T0124304

CHRONIC PAIN:
A Self-Help Guide

A Two-Part Book of My Journey
with Chronic Pain

AND

Part 2:
A Self-Help Guide for
Coping with Chronic Pain

STEVEN W. POLLARD, PHD

Chronic Pain:

A Self-Help Guide

Chronic Pain:
A Self-Help Guide

A Two-Part Book of My Journey with
Chronic Pain and Part 2: A Self-Help
Guide for Coping with Chronic Pain

Steven W. Pollard, PhD

iUniverse, Inc.
Bloomington

Chronic Pain: A Self-Help Guide
A Two-Part Book of My Journey with Chronic Pain and
Part 2: A Self-Help Guide for Coping with Chronic Pain

iUniverse books may be ordered through booksellers or by contacting:

iUniverse
1663 Liberty Drive
Bloomington, IN 47403
www.iuniverse.com
1-800-Authors (1-800-288-4677)

Because of the dynamic nature of the Internet, any web addresses or links contained in this book may have changed since publication and may no longer be valid. The views expressed in this work are solely those of the author and do not necessarily reflect the views of the publisher, and the publisher hereby disclaims any responsibility for them.

Any people depicted in stock imagery provided by Thinkstock are models, and such images are being used for illustrative purposes only.
Certain stock imagery © Thinkstock.

Library of Congress Control Number: 2011909739

ISBN: 978-1-4620-3034-7 (pbk)
ISBN: 978-1-4620-3035-4 (ebk)

Printed in the United States of America

iUniverse rev. date: 06/27/2011

CONTENTS

Endorsements

Tom Catton

Author of *The Mindful Addict: A Memoir of the Awakening of a Spirit*

Chronic Pain by Steven Pollard, PhD, is a must read for those experiencing chronic pain, and I might add even more of a must read for the doctors who treat patients with chronic pain.

I found this book difficult to read because of the brutal honesty within the pages. It made me grateful that I don't have chronic pain and somewhat fearful of the thought that this can happen to anyone simply by bending over to pick up a newspaper.

Steven W. Pollard, PhD

This is a self-help book of Steven's own chronic pain. The book is so compelling because the words were not born of theory or study in the area of chronic pain, but from someone whose life has been severely interrupted with this daily challenge. Steven takes us on his journey along the complex road of his pain. We experience the powerlessness he feels when going from one source to the next for healing that never seems to come, the hope that is extinguished with every new visit, the frustration of dealing with insurance companies, doctors who seem to almost give up when they realize they can't heal, and disappointment when he attempts certain alternative practices. This excursion will provide us with as close an understanding as one can have without trudging the road of being a chronic-pain victim.

This book is not meant to be a feel-good adventure, but it will touch the reader's heart and may reveal to a doctor, or caregiver, or family member a new level of compassion in the area of chronic pain.

From Perry, one of my chronic-pain patients.

"I'm replying to your honest and brilliant work of pain self-help. Your truthfulness throughout all chapters has provided me ways in helping me cope with my pain. As with you, a lot of what is mentioned is what I've had and been experiencing over the past and present. I recommend you don't remove the cuss words when publishing your book. There are those people who have pain but then there are people with f***ing pain who are those who can relate with your book. Those who study pain have no true knowledge of pain; they only have an idea of what pain is like. Sometimes I like to park by the airport and yell and cuss as loud and louder than the jets that are taking off for therapy myself. Well, I'd like to thank *You* Dr. Pollard for providing me with all your professionalism and honesty of what it's like to live with pain. You're a hero and a scholar in my book and as you said, for others as well."

Steven W. Pollard, PhD

Greg Ruhland, MD
Pain-Management Specialist: Hilo, Hawaii

In the story of his personal self-help with pain, Dr. Pollard has poignantly documented the intricacies of living with a chronic disease. It is a story for patients with chronic pain, their families, and health-care providers. It is a tale of life transition from a healthy semi-retired psychologist to a full-time patient with severe, chronic pain. The paradox—Dr. Pollard treated patients with chronic-pain syndrome for many years in his private practice and therefore has a unique perspective of this condition. This is the best resource I have seen regarding this often-devastating condition.

PART ONE:

Dear reader, if you find errors such as typos, misspelling, poor grammar, and/or punctuation, please forgives me. This is not the fault of the publisher but rather my own as I chose not to have them do a re-edit and a final proof read to catch such errors. I hope that you won't let that distract you from reading and benefiting from the contents of the book.

Chapter I:
Death

I Want to Die. The original title of this book was "Dead Life: Life Dead" but some of my friends said it sounded too gloomy. And well, I didn't really want to die but at times I really did want to die. I just couldn't go on living that way. Rather, I didn't and don't want to live with this pain. When you have severe, chronic pain it is like being dead.

Well, no, really, sometimes I really want to die to escape the pain and the loss of quality of life that results from it. It's like living in a cesspool of human waste similar to the "Slum Dog Millionaire." This all sounds confusing and reflects the confused state of mind that comes with chronic, severe pain. F*** it.

How did I get here? Who'd have thought that my life would end up like this? F*** this shit.

Dear reader, I apologize for my vulgarity here and in other parts of this book. I don't generally curse but sometimes that is the only way to express the feelings I have, to break through the polite circle of courteous behavior. Severe pain doesn't give a f*** about politeness. Intense continuous pain, tears, and rages. Rage at the pain, the "system" that supposedly treats it, and how the pain goes on and on, and never stops. When my patients read it, they say, "Yeah. Doc. You really know what it's like. The cursing has to stay in the book cause that's what makes it real. It makes me feel like I can talk to you. You get it. Leave the curse words in; they make the book seem more real."

So why should you buy and read this book? Because it's about learning how to cope with the pain. This self-book is for people who suffer unbearable, severe, screaming bad pain and those who live with, love, and support them. In spite of the pain they continue to live, as much as they can, sometimes a breath at a time, looking at the sky, seeing the clouds, feeling the cool breeze and the warm sun, and gradually build a new life out of the catastrophe of their pain, even though the pain never goes away. Chronic pain happens—it is real. You have to deal with it. You have no choice. Suffering is, however, to some degree, optional. It is very difficult if not impossible to get across to someone who doesn't have or who hasn't had severe, chronic pain, how totally, totally devastating, debilitating, debasing, and humiliating it is. It is like being dead but alive or alive but dead in all the things you used to be able to do; simple things like bending down to tie a shoe, or opening a door, or even getting out of bed. It takes me an hour or two to get up and going. First I wake up, and then I think about moving my body and getting my legs off the bed, and then sitting for a few minutes to get the energy to actually stand up. Then there is the slow walk to the bathroom, then brushing my teeth and squatting down so that I don't lean over the sink—as that simple act of bending over will cause me more pain.

I've read other books on chronic pain, supposedly written by persons with chronic pain, but their description of their pain doesn't come close to coming through in their written words. They either haven't really had severe, chronic pain, or they are missing the point by trying to make it an academic review of research.

By sharing my story I hope to let you know that you aren't alone and that there are some things you can do to decrease the suffering. There is water in the desert; you just have to find out how to get it. My story of my own pain and suffering also lets you know that I have been there, am there, which I hope will make my suggestions of self-help more meaningful to you. I have worked with more than a hundred chronic severe pain patients, and I have learned more from them than from any textbook or course for treating Chronic Pain.

I purposely do not cite many sources, as this is not meant to be an academic work. I have tried each of the specific strategies mention and found that some worked for me and some didn't. I caution you and urge you to consult your MD before trying any of the coping skills I suggest.

For those who are interested I have many academic credentials as follows:

PROFESSIONAL ORGANIZATIONS:

Member: American Psychological Association (APA)
American Society of Clinical Hypnosis
National Register of Health Service Providers in Psychology
Hawaii Psychological Association (prior Board Member)
Hawaii Island Psychological Association
Association for the Treatment of Sex Abusers
Continuing Education/Peer Review Group (Hilo)

Diplomate: The American Board of Forensic Examiners
The American Board of Forensic Medicine
The American Board of Disability Analysts
The American Board of Psychological Specialties in Child Psychology

Certificate:	of Proficiency from APA in treatment of Alcohol and Drug abuse (not current)
	Certificate of Professional Qualification in Psychology (State & Provincial Psychology Boards)
Professional:	Consulting Editor for "Forensic Psychology and Neuropsychology for Criminal and Civil Cases" CRC Press 2008

Before using any of my suggestions I again strongly recommend and even insist that you consult with you own MD.

I was strongly influenced by "Anatomy of Illness" by Norman Cousins in his description of his pain and his journey back to health. I also relied on information from "Mind as Healer, Mind as Slayer" by Kenneth R. Pelletier

One of the reasons that chronic pain is so hard to treat is that each person's pain is different and responds differently to various treatments. What may work for one patient won't work for anther, or what works for a while quits working after some months.

Chapter 2:
Stages of Pain

I've come to think of pain as having stages, much like those of grief. First comes denial, then anger, bartering, depression, and finally acceptance. However, these don't occur in a linear fashion one after the other or in a straight line. They occur in a mixed-up order and the stages aren't static; that is, one doesn't finish with one stage and never go back to it. You might be in all five stages at once and/or you might go from one to the other and back in one day or one hour. It's like being a boxer in a ring full of dozens of other fighters all punching you repeatedly and it seems that there is no way out.

To me, grief for a lost loved one is easier to cope with as it—the death—is over, and time does lessen the pain for most people. Chronic physical-emotional pain is never over; it goes on and on, hour after hour, day after day, week after week, month after month, like the fires of hell never go out. You get the picture.

I use the hyphenated word physical-emotional pain, as all chronic physical pain has at least some, and usually a lot, of emotional trauma. Of course the reverse can also be true—that emotional hurt can cause physical pain. However, that doesn't make the pain any less real: more on this later in the section on "Types of Pain."

Denial

It isn't that you deny having pain, but you/I deny that it is not going away and has become chronic. This is much more insidious than that, however. It's the denial of the reality that you can't do even the simple things you used to be able to do, like unloading the dishwasher, bending down to pick up a dropped paper, playing on the floor with a child, or any of the things that you could do prior to having the pain: the creeping loss of independence. "This isn't happening to me. I'm stronger than this." Having to depend on others for simple things like driving to appointments and not being able to go to evening events without someone to drive you because you're on so much medication you can't drive. All of this pain and medications erodes your very soul like a trickle of water that eventually erodes the earth and causes deep furrows and even deeper gullies of despair.

This stage is very vicious as it causes a self-destructive circle of trying to do things you deny that you can't do, then doing them and suffering the consequent aggravated, severe pain. I kept asking myself, "What did I do to make my pain worse? I didn't do anything." But I had done something.

One time I had simply kayaked out to my son's sailboat and stood and sat and watched him work on his boat. Kayaking is just like paddling a small canoe. I can kayak because I have good lumbar support and am not in pain as long as I don't stay in the same position too long. I can do lots of things like walking and riding my stationary bike without any pain: more on this later. What I can't do is stand still for more than a few minutes, or sit in one position too long, or lie on my back for too long.

I just watched my son work and swayed with the boat's movements. But that evening my pain was much worse. The kayak paddling time to the boat was only 10 minutes. Surely I could do that? Before my chronic pain I had been riding a stationary bike almost daily for sixty to ninety minutes. Since my injury I have continued to ride but not as much. But standing and sitting in the swaying boat did cause my back to hurt the next day. No more kayaking, at least for a while. Or maybe it wasn't the kayaking. Balancing myself with the gentle rocking of the boat puts lots of minor repetitive stress on the back. The pain is like small threads of a fine garment that are pulled out one at a time, almost unnoticed until the bare pain is exposed.

Another time I had to get a new refrigerator. I unloaded the old one and after the new one was delivered I loaded it with the stuff from the old one. A very simple task, nothing over three lbs. or so, and not very much of that, but again I was in severe pain afterwards. It was like Sisyphus pushing the dung ball up the hill only to have it roll back down and he'd have to start over again, on and on.

How many times do I have to keep re-injuring my back and exacerbating the pain? How many times did Sisyphus have to push his load up the hill? Forever. Why do I keep denying that I can't do even these simple things? The answer is simply that to admit that I can't do these things is admitting that I'm helpless and dependent on others. I know intellectually that we are all dependent on others for different things at different times, but to go from being able to do most everything for oneself, to not being able to do most anything is something I didn't want to admit. Hence: the denial. I have to remind myself that there are many things that I can do and that I'm not helpless—I can talk, walk, ride my bike, and go places during the day.

I was in aquatherapy one day and saw a man enter in a motorized wheelchair and the assistant helped him from his chair into a crane type of chair that could then lower him into the heated water of the pool. There were only about three of us in the pool at that time and I told him I admired him and that it made me feel good. I hadn't put it correctly and he said, "Well if my being in a wheelchair makes you happy then good for you." I hastily tried to correct my comments. I admired him for doing what he could and not giving up. What made me happy was his effort despite his handicaps and I was thankful that I didn't have a situation as bad as his. If he could do it I had no excuse to quit trying to handle my own pain. My happiness was for his inspiration.

I have had to get past the denial and admit my limitations. But it has not been easy and I still deny some limitations even to myself. But I'm learning. Pain is an exacting teacher. The furrows and gullies of pain are still there.

I am a clinical psychologist and have been in private practice for 37 years. One of my pain patients told me how much she used to enjoy going to the mall and walking around and watching all the people, but now she couldn't engage in even this simple pleasure due to her pain. She couldn't walk for more than a few paces and then had to sit down. She refused to use a wheelchair. She was too ashamed to admit that she was in pain—but not because she wanted to be. Unfortunately, she saw her life as her failure, to be unable to walk. She felt guilty about it, concerned that when others would see her they would pity her or think she was making it up.

Thankfully I've gotten past that guilt trap. When I need a wheelchair, for example, going through an art exhibit or an airport, I ask for one and use it, but I understand her loss of pride.

Anger/Fear/Hurt

Anger is easier to understand. Of course I'm angry and so would you be. If someone hit you in the head, or leg, or back with a baseball bat, you'd hurt too. It hurts Goddamn it, it hurts f***ing bad and it doesn't quit. I'm angry at the pain, at the need for medication, and for being so overly dependent on others. I fear what will happen to me next. I finally get a medication combination that seems to give me some relief, but my constant fear is: "What if the doctor won't give me anymore?" or, "My God, how can I live without this medication?" The pain hurts so bad. I've got to have the medication. I'll just hammer the son of a bitch if he won't give me the prescription; let him see what the pain feels like. Why the hell can't I f***ing bend over and pick things up? I've done things like that all my life.

What the f*** does that doctor know about pain? They want me to get off the narcotics because they are addictive. Fine if they can give me an alternative that works. If not, f*** them. I'd rather be addicted than in so much pain.

The anger goes on and is directed at any thing or person that happens to be near at hand; a spouse, a friend, or a stranger. Any small thing can set you over the edge—just someone asking an innocent question like "How are you?" or saying, "Have a nice day." It's like a huge dam of water that's constantly about to break over the top and drown the victims below the dam.

One of the first functions that should be taught to service personnel, or to anyone living with a person in chronic pain, is to ask them if they are in pain, and if so, to give them a chance to cool down, and not to ask them again.

Of course the anger leads to guilt for having snapped at someone close to you or even to strangers who simply may have said "Good day." A little of the water had spilled over the dam. And the guilt makes the pain worse. It is another vicious circle, the more the pain, the more the anger, which makes you tense, which makes the pain worse, which makes you more angry and/or depressed, and you end up feeling helpless, useless, and hopeless. Anger has been called a camouflage emotion because usually it is really covering up hurt. It's, to some degree, like being tied down on a torture rack with each person turning the wheel stretching you out and causing you more agony.

Depression

These feelings of helplessness and hopelessness are symptoms of depression. Part of depression is the denial that one is depressed. I denied that I was/am depressed. I had/have suicidal thoughts but "I'm NOT depressed." The fact that my sleep was disturbed, I was gaining weight—from eating comfort foods—and that I would start crying for the least reason, were simply from the pain. I was isolating myself, because I didn't want to bring other people down with my moaning and groaning. If I didn't have the pain, I wouldn't have any of those symptoms, so "I'm NOT depressed, I'm in pain. GET IT? I'm NOT depressed." (Denial is more than a river in Egypt.)

Okay, okay. I'm depressed. I'll take the f***ing medication. And then we're back to anger. And so it goes, round and round. Side effects of medications will be discussed later.

The feeling of helplessness and hopelessness is like what happens to laboratory rats. If they are held in a gloved hand until they quit struggling and then placed in a bucket of water with high sides, they almost immediately drown. Whereas a rat who hasn't been held in a hand until it quits struggling and is placed immediately in the same bucket of water will keep on swimming for hours before it drowns.

Some patients I see readily admit that they are depressed, some deny it like I did, and some aren't even aware that they are depressed. It's one of the standard questions in therapy: "Are you depressed and if so where would you place yourself on a 1-10 scale of depression?"

Bartering

This occurs on many levels concerning medications, activities, religion, and others. For example: "Can't I have some stronger medication? I'll do the physical therapy, if you'll just give me something stronger." Or, "It's been three hours since my last pain pill. So I can take another one now even though it's supposed to be every four hours. Taking it one hour sooner won't hurt. Besides, no one will know." Or, "God, let me get through this play tonight and I promise I will limit myself to two beers, only two, please, please. I want to see my daughter's performance."

Acceptance

God, this is the difficult part. Will Sisyphus ever get the ball up to the top of the hill without it rolling back down? Accepting that I'm disabled; that I can't work, can't do the things that I used to do; that I have to ask others to help me, and I fear that I have and will always have this pounding pain that never goes away except for a little while. This is not the way I want to live. I hope I can find ways to live around the pain.

Or, as I say to my patients sometimes, "Your mission—from the old show 'Mission Impossible'—should you choose to accept it, Mr. Phelps, is to build a life larger than your pain, a life different from your past life." I and my patients need, and this is absolutely critical, to accept the mission of building a different life that includes pain, and limitations, and new possibilities, and a meaning and purpose to our lives. Without this we return to the hopeless, helpless life of despair and suffering. Sisyphus needs to leave the ball at the bottom of the hill and build a new life around it.

Chapter 3:
The Argument for Living

There are many reasons to choose to live rather than to kill yourself. Number one is that if the pain gets and stays too unbearable you can always go back to this option. But once you've done this one, there is no going back, undo, or do over.

What seems unbearable now may become less so as time goes on. Most people don't like beer when they first taste it but as time goes on with more drinking they learn to love it. One of the things that make physical pain worse is the way you interpret it. Studies of pain patients during World War II found that patients with the same severity of wounds required different amounts of pain medication depending on the meaning they attached to the pain. Patients who were munitions' factory workers on the mainland, with wives and children, who had an industrial accident that crushed their legs, would require two to three times as much pain medication as compared to soldiers on the front line in Germany with similarly severe wounds.

What's the difference? Both groups of patients had identical wounds. The difference—in addition to individual differences in response to pain—was the meaning that the pain had for the patients. For the factory worker it meant the loss of his job, no ability to pay his mortgage or feed his family, and that he was a failure. For the soldier, the pain meant he had the "million-dollar wound." The loss of his leg meant he would live and be sent home to start his new life. Sisyphus had quit trying to push the ball up the hill.

What's the message here? It is how you interpret the meaning of the pain that, to a large degree, determines not only how much pain medication you need, but also how much you suffer.

As Kermit the frog would say, "It ain't easy being green." Having severe, chronic pain is not easy. It's one of the most difficult things in life to cope with, especially chronic pain that others can't "see." For most chronic-pain patients the pain means loss of function, loss of job, and loss of the ability to do almost all of the things they were used to doing. They have a *Dead Life* or are like the living dead.

So what is the argument for living? There is the religious one, but I'm not going into that one, although I encourage you to do that if that is helpful for you. There is the fact that the pain may bring you to new experiences in life that you would not have had without the pain. John McCain said, with all sincerity, that he was grateful for his POW torture experience—which obviously was very painful for him—because without it he wouldn't be the person he became in order to run for President of the United States of America in 2008.

Killing yourself has only one positive—and that is the end of suffering for you. But it causes huge amounts of suffering for the loved ones you leave behind. First, try to see if you can find some ways of decreasing the suffering. Again, pain is not optional, but suffering is.

It REALLY ain't easy.

Chapter 4:
Types of Pain

There are obviously many types of pain. There is physical pain caused by some disorder of the body that will show up in various tests such as blood chemistry, CAT scans, MRIs, X-rays, and others. Unfortunately, there are many, many people who have real pain but there is nothing wrong with the body—at least as far as these medical tests indicate. That doesn't mean that the pain isn't real or that it is caused by emotional problems. It only means that the current state of medical science, or art, is not sufficiently refined enough to identify the source of the pain.

A single nerve from an infected tooth may cause excruciating pain but it would not necessarily show up on any of the tests mentioned. The only evidence of the pain is the patient's statement of feelings of pain. Understandably, many doctors get frustrated when they can't find any physical evidence of the cause of the pain, and then when the standard treatments for the pain don't work, they conclude that it's an emotional problem, or that the patient is making it up for some reason.

I have had almost all the medical tests that can be done and have consulted with four separate pain specialists as well as my primary care physician (PCP). They all reach the same conclusion: that there is no physical evidence of the cause of my pain. One of my later MRIs did show some "mild degenerative disk disorder." It is the doctors' consensus that I need to take my pain medication, and learn to live with it, and that it might get better with time. They liken my pain to an athletic injury where the muscle and/or ligaments are torn and will take time to heal. However, there are no physical findings to explain my pain.

I get comments that my symptoms are very unusual. My pain is located in my lower lumbar back (L4 and L5) and doesn't radiate down or up. It doesn't keep me from walking, riding my stationary bike (more about this later), or climbing stairs. I can bend over but, if I do, or do it repeatedly, the pain gets much worse.

I can't stand in one place for more than a few minutes, or sit for more than twenty minutes without having severe pain. As the day goes on my pain becomes worse. If I lie flat on my back for more than an hour my pain used to become worse. Now however, it is like being in heaven to lie on a hot pad with a rolled-up towel under my lower back with a towel on top of the heating pad.

My pain was not caused by any accident or work injury. I'm not suing anyone and have no secondary gain—money or special attention—from the pain.

Other patients who have pains that can't be explained by the physical evidence often get misdiagnosed as having some sort of emotional problem, specifically depression and/or a psychosomatic disorder; that is, the source of the pain is some emotional problem that is expressed through the physical symptoms of pain. Yes, the patient is depressed, but it is the pain that is causing the depression, not the depression causing the pain. However, depression does make pain worse.

Psychosomatic pain or emotional trauma that causes physical pain does exist. A person may have a heart attack that looks just like a real heart attack on the electrocardiogram (EKG) but other tests don't show any blocked arteries or clogged blood vessels. The heart, which is a muscle, spasms like a Charlie Horse leg cramp. The cause for this type of heart attack may be extreme stress and/or anger. There is some truth to the homily that "He died of a broken heart." Men sometimes experience "labor pains" along with their wives.

The fact that some people do suffer from psychosomatic pain makes it especially difficult for patients who are on "Workman's Compensation" or who were in some kind of accident and are suing for damages. In these cases, where there is some money involved, many physicians, erroneously, conclude that the pain is exaggerated, psychosomatic, and/or due to some pre-existing condition or life trauma, such as an alcoholic parent. If there is no physical evidence supporting the patient's pain symptoms, then the patient must be making it up. The absence or lack of evidence of physical disease is not evidence that physical disease doesn't exist. The state of medical science is not advanced enough yet to see the evidence. You can't see electricity but it is there—just stick your finger in the light socket and turn on the switch. (No, don't do that.) It's like telling a man who is dying of dehydration that he doesn't need to drink any water. What—are you nuts? Yes many MDs are nuts.

In my experience, none of the patients I have treated for chronic pain are exaggerating their symptoms or making them up. Many, in fact, under-report their symptoms, trying to be tough and/or polite. These patients really want to go back to work and their pain-free life, yet they can't, due to the pain and/or the emotional trauma that comes with the pain. Unfortunately, they are lumped in the same diagnostic category as those who do have true psychosomatic pain. My diagnoses of patients are based on seeing the patient on numerous occasions, twenty to sixty or more times, seeing their significant others, and talking to their other treating MDs.

I admit that I probably have a skewed sample of chronic-pain patients, as I doubt that any patient making the symptoms up would go to see a psychologist.

Chapter 5:
How I Got Here

So how did I get here and who am I to write a self-help book about my pain? I had a story to tell that had the potential to help millions of chronic-pain suffers and their families. I'm certainly no hero and there are millions of others who suffer far more severely than I do. So why do I write this: to share my "story" with others in the hope that some parts of it will help them with their pain. This is also part of my own treatment.

I'm 68 and a semi-retired clinical psychologist and part-time abstract artist and writer. That means I see patients two days a week and do a half-day of "paper" administrative work to keep the office going. I'm a solo practitioner and so do most everything myself. At the time my pain really began, I was in reasonably good health, 5 foot 7 inches tall, and my weight had been stable for about four years at 175 lbs.

My journey into pain all began very innocently back in October of 2007 when a fellow abstract artist asked me if I'd help him "flesh in" the character of a psychologist in one of his novels. I said yes and began spending hours bent over my computer keyboard typing dialogue. It was as though my thoughts went straight from my brain to my fingers on the keyboard, like turning on a faucet and the water just flows out. Hours would go by. I was having fun. I'd go sometimes three or four hours typing and not moving from my chair. Then when I did get up my back would be sore, so I'd stretch for a few minutes and then go back to typing. I did this for days and weeks at a time.

When my colleague decided he didn't want to use my "character" in his book, I decided to write my own book. While in the process, I would complain from time to time to my daughter about my back hurting and she'd say, "Well, you really need to stretch dad." That was very good advice. But I was having so much fun building my characters that I often forgot.

About the end of October, 2007, I took a planned vacation to visit a friend on the mainland. When I got there I was a zombie, from being up all night and stuck in a metal tube for the 14-hour plane trip from Hilo, Hawaii. Luckily, I had some "pain" meds, *Lyrica* and *Neurotin*—more about these later—and my back got somewhat better. We had a good visit that lasted about 10 days before I headed back to Hilo, where I returned to seeing my patients and writing my novel.

At that time I was seeing patients three-to-four and a half days a week. I was also doing some digital painting to get ready for a "solo" on-line abstract art show and for a couple of local competitions. I wasn't writing as much, but when I did my back was still trying to tell me to stop. I finished my first draft and set the book aside for most of November and December. Then I got back to writing and did a second draft and edited it word by word, line by line. By now my back was seriously hurting, and I finally took my daughter's advice and started stretching every hour. I had to set a kitchen timer to remind me when to stop, which I did, but then I'd just reset the timer and go back to writing and/or editing.

By January or February of 2008 my back was hurting so much it was interfering with my ability to sleep. So I contacted my MD and, in addition to *Ambien*, he prescribed some hydorcodone for the pain. I couldn't take many muscle relaxants as I was on *Warfaren*—a blood thinner—from a previous deep-vein thrombosis problem. The doctor also had me get an X-ray, a CAT scan, and an MRI, the results of which were all "normal." That was the good news: there was nothing overtly abnormal with my spine which could explain the pain. The bad news was that I still had the severe pain which was getting worse. I had to quit seeing patients at 5 PM and then at 4 as, by that time of the day, I was in so much pain I couldn't stop the tears from streaming down my face.

I had tried many of the home remedies suggested by numerous people. Various types of stretching, Kava tea to relax, heating pads, cold pads, and almost anything anyone suggested to me. It was like giving an electrician water or paint brushes to fix an electrical problem. Nothing seemed to really help and it was getting to be very annoying, so I scheduled another appointment with my doctor, a family practitioner.

My pain was like a heavy, dull ache right on the spine in the low back, L4 and L5 area. That's the small curved area just above your tailbone. Many of my other lack of symptoms, he said—and I agreed—were very unusual for back pain. The pain didn't radiate out at all; it was mostly gone in the morning but got worse as the day wore on. Lying down at night on my back was the worst at that time. Later in my journey of pain, lying down on my bed with a rolled up towel under the hot pad (placed in the L4-L5 area) and a towel on top provided the most relief. On a 1-to-10 scale—which is the way almost all pain clinics have you rate your pain—with 10 being excruciating, screaming, unbearable pain, I rated it at 6 or 7 at its worst. The pain didn't keep me from doing much of anything; I walked up and down several flights of stairs several times a day, rode my stationary bike almost every day for 30 to 45 minutes, and went kayaking occasionally. None of this physical activity made the pain worse, in fact, riding the bike made me feel better, but I always did that in the mornings. As the day wore on, typically my back began to hurt more. If I sat too long or stood still for more than a few minutes it would begin to hurt unbearably.

I muddled along for a few more weeks but the pain was getting worse—of course I was still typing and editing my "novel." I remembered that I had a friend who was a pain-management specialist MD and called him for an appointment. He tried some "facet injections" and when that made it worse, he tried some epidural injections, which also made it worse. He also prescribed *Lyrica* and *Neurontin* to "quiet down" the nerve impulses that were sending the pain signals to my conscious brain. They didn't help.

By the time pain has become chronic, it's like an 8-lane highway carrying the pain symptoms to the conscious brain but only one lane of messages back to the pain area to relax.

Chapter 6:
The Pain Weekend

On a Thursday towards the end of April of 2008 my pain was really bad, especially at night. That night I had taken four hydrocodone pills, though I was only prescribed two a day. I hadn't slept all night and I had gotten constipated to the point of severe constipation pain, which is often a side effect of pain medications, especially the opiates like hydrocodone, *Oxycontin*, morphine, and others. It was like someone sticking a broomstick up your butt. Friday morning I called my MD but they were closed for the weekend. So I went to the "Urgent Care Center" and was honest with them when they asked me if my pain was on-going. I said yes, and they said that they could only treat acute back pain and couldn't do anything for my constipation—which by then was worse than my back pain. I knew that I wouldn't get any help from the emergency room and it would mean painful waiting for several hours for no help. It's like telling a person with a punctured lung to take a deep breath. Yeah, right.

I went to my local drug store and got some *Fleet* enemas, which had been suggested by the Urgent Care Center. I had asked the pharmacist if they had anything I could take orally that would be quicker than the several hours that a laxative would take. He said no. That is not true; there are some prescription medications that I could have taken and I could have been advised to try suppositories.

The *Fleet* enemas provided very little relief, but by the next day the laxative had worked. But that night I was in severe pain sitting on the side of my bed and rocking back and forth and moaning. I knew I couldn't go on with my life like that. That Saturday and Sunday I continued to suffer and take pain pills and laxatives.

Cannabis

Sometime in May 2008 I applied for my "Medical Cannabis License." This involved an in-depth interview by a local MD who specializes in this area. He also reviewed my medical records from my other treating doctors.

I had heard from many of the chronic-pain patients that I see in my practice that smoking a joint would greatly relieve the pain. Fortunately, the State of Hawaii has legalized the medical use of cannabis. Of course, Federal law nullifies State law, even though there are several other states which have legalized the medical use of cannabis. Notwithstanding this Federal trump of State law, Federal officials don't usually prosecute cannabis users who have a legitimate state license to use cannabis for medical treatment. In Hawaii several years ago there was a big case about Federal prosecutors seizing pot plants from three chronic-pain patients, who had medical cannabis licenses, and they were prosecuting them for cannabis abuse. It was a huge story and pictures of the Federal officials and the three arrested individuals with their pot plants were shown on the front page of the local paper with headlines about the arrests. Three or four days later there was an equally big story about the Federal prosecutors dropping the charges, apologizing to the patients, and even giving back the confiscated plants. If one is using or growing cannabis beyond the amount allowed by the State law, they may indeed need to fear prosecution from Federal prosecutors, and there is no guarantee that they won't be prosecuted anyway.

The law in Hawaii has some quirks in it. The MD who certified that I met the criteria to have a license explained to me that he couldn't tell me how to get any. He did give me information about the law in Hawaii. I could have up to seven plants, four mature and three seedlings, and up to three ounces of dried cannabis buds.

He did give me the name of someone I could contact on the Internet who could advise me. I met with that person after calling him on the phone. He gave me all kinds of literature on how to grow cannabis. Even when I'm not confused by pain and pain medications, every thing I have ever tried to grow has died, and I knew I couldn't do all the "growing" procedures he was recommending.

By word of mouth I was able to find a source. The Hawaii law makes it legal—at the State level—for me to buy and have cannabis, but illegal for anyone to sell it to me. Yeah, that's what I said. It's like saying you can drink water if you can find some but it is illegal for anyone to sell you any water.

Now that I had some cannabis I wondered how I should use it. I didn't have any cigarette papers to roll my own and I really didn't want to smoke it anyway, as I don't smoke. I vaguely remembered taking a "toke" or two in graduate school. I had gotten a copy of *High Times*, which is a magazine dedicated to cannabis growing and using. The first night I had some I didn't know what to do but was able to figure it out. Smoking it is quick but bad for your lungs. I really don't know how people smoke pot and go to work. I only smoked it in the evening before bed and only three to four tokes a night. That is enough to get rid of the pain but it leaves me totally dysfunctional; I couldn't walk a straight line much less drive anywhere. Since one of the "expert" MDs I was seeing at the time told me I had to quit or they wouldn't be able to prescribe the narcotics, I have quit. I never smoked it to "get high", but I do remember times when everything was very funny for no reason.

Chapter 7:

On-Going Journey: Chop Wood, Carry Water

After that "pain weekend", on Monday I went to see my regular MD for an urgent appointment. When he entered the inner examination room, where his nurse had put me, I was on my hands and knees doing the cat exercise of arching my back up and then bending my stomach towards the floor. It was the only way I could manage the pain. That appointment was at the end of the day and I was exhausted from the pain. You know how it is with MD visits—you don't know how long you'll have to wait in the inner exam room before you actually see the doctor.

I was embarrassed to have been caught on the floor. He asked what was wrong. I just started bawling, the tears flowing down my cheeks.

The floodgate of my damned-up feelings had been broken. Through my tears I said, "I'm in pain."

He said, "Are you taking the pain meds I prescribed?"

"No," I said.

"Why not?" he asked.

"Because I don't want to be a druggy," I cried through my tears that were still streaming down my face.

He gave me a *Kleenex* and I gradually recovered my composure. I told him how I had seen so many patients who used and abused drugs and I didn't want to get labeled as a "drug-seeking" patient.

He told me to take the hydrocodone up to four a day and *Oxycodone* one-to-two times a day for "break-out pain." I thanked him through tears and took the prescriptions to a local drug store. I left them with the pharmacy and went to run some errands, as it always takes them a couple of hours to fill a prescription. When I came back to the drug store they told me they didn't carry *Oxycodone* so I had to take it to another pharmacy across town. This may sound like minor stuff to you, but when you're in pain it's a big deal. It's like telling someone with profuse bleeding that you can't treat that here and you'll have to go across town to get treatment.

Over the next several months I tried a variety of treatments. My pain-management specialist again gave me a series of facet shots in the outer layer of the spinal area. He and his assistant gave me a drug "cocktail", a local anesthetic, prior to the procedure so that the procedure wouldn't hurt, but when these medications had worn off the pain was worse. So a few weeks later, the doctor tried more injections, this time into the epidural area of the spine. Again, once the medications that I took for the procedure of the shots wore off, the pain was worse.

In the meantime I was continuing on the hydrocodone and *Oxycodone* during the day with *Ambien, Neurontin, Lyrica,* and a muscle relaxant at bedtime and was managing semi-okay. I may have the sequence of these things somewhat mixed up but they all occurred. My grown daughter and my former wife—who both lived in the same town as me—had started accompanying me, at my request, to my medical appointments. I was very grateful for their help as I had trouble remembering what was said and I wanted to keep things straight. Also I wanted the doctors to know that I wasn't going from one doctor to the next trying to get drugs.

My friend, the pain-management specialist, was honest and said he didn't know anything else to do and he referred me to another MD in town who did some pain management similar to his. This doctor suggested some "Prolotherapy" spinal shots—essentially injecting a sugar solution into the ligaments. This type of therapy usually took three or more times of being injected before getting significant relief. Since this is considered experimental and not in the mainstream of medicine, my health insurance wouldn't cover the injections.

This doctor's reasoning sounded good. She said that my injury was like a sports' injury when the muscles, tendons, and ligaments get injured and that it may take six months to several years to heal. I decided to try it. She didn't believe in "drug cocktails" but did offer me 10 mg of *Valium*. I was in tears in her office and at first I said no to the *Valium* but then quickly changed my mind and said, "Fuck it. Give me the *Valium*." I was tired of the hurting. She did, and after waiting some time for the *Valium* to kick in, she then proceeded to give me the shots. I used my charge card for the payment of $250.

The doctor had said to keep track of the pain and to rate it daily, and that we'd know in three to four weeks whether or not it would work. My hopes were up.

Three or four weeks later I went back and told her my pain was worse, if anything. She said, that being the case, she couldn't recommend continuing with any more of the injections. At least she didn't charge me for that session.

On the same day that I had my initial appointment for consultation about the Prolotherapy shots, I tried acupuncture. I had some time before that consultation and was walking around where I had parked. I saw a sign in front of a building that said "Acupuncture." It was in mid-afternoon and my back was beginning to hurt. I walked up some stairs to the office and asked some questions about the process, and said I thought that I'd like to try it. The woman said, "How about now?"

"Okay," I said.

She took me back to a room that had two curtained partitions and a massage table in each. She had me undress to my underwear and gave me a towel to put over me. When she came back I was lying on the table on my back, and she asked me to turn over on my stomach, and then she put acupuncture needles in various parts of my body, arms, hands, legs, feet, ears, back, and head.

She left me to lie still for what seemed like about 10 or 15 minutes. There was soothing soft music playing on speakers. When she came back she took out the needles and had me lie on my back, and again inserted needles in various places. Fifteen minutes later she came back again and removed the needles, and told me to take my time and get up when I felt like it.

I was amazed. My pain was gone!

I walked to the front of her office and paid her $40 cash and she said, "Oh, by the way my name is . . ."

"I'm Steve," I said.

By early that evening the pain was back. It wasn't until I thought about it that evening that I realized that there was something wrong with what had happened. She didn't take any history, or ask me any questions, or have me sign anything. She did give me a business card that said she was licensed. But there was absolutely no proof that I had ever been there. There was no written record and I had paid her in cash—cash or check were the only options. She didn't even know my full name. Somehow I felt it was unprofessional and I didn't go back. I didn't get around to trying another acupuncturist for a long time, and when I did it I went five times and it would feel better for an hour or two. At $45 per 30-minute session I didn't think it was worth it as the pain always came back. I did get some cream to rub on the area of pain: "*Somba* pain gell." It goes on cold but then heats up with body heat. This worked well but if you put it on too often it causes a rash, or, it did for me, so I couldn't use it too often. You can find it on-line. If you try it make sure that you don't get any in your eyes or genital areas.

During the next several months I had referrals to three different physical therapists. The first one was a combination of a chiropractic and physical therapist (PT). She did a verbal assessment of my symptoms, which almost all professionals do, and that makes my recitation of symptoms seem flat from having told them so often. She then did some manipulation and had an assistant who did some "Shiatsu-like" massage of "trigger points" on my spine. At first she was kind of gentle and then as she pushed more deeply it hurt some. She asked my permission to "go for it" and I said yes, not really knowing what to expect. Her thumbs dug deep into those trigger spots on my back and I was screaming out loud, and several people put their heads in to see what was going on. "I asked you if it was okay to 'go for it,'" she said.

I just groaned and she must have taken that as my permission to continue and I guess I did want her to, as it felt so good when she would let up in between pushing on the trigger points. When she was finished I had to admit that the pain was gone! WOW. What a relief. But it was more like hitting your thumb with a hammer so that you won't notice the pain in your back.

I was pain free! I couldn't believe it. Unfortunately, it only lasted about four or five hours. After the third session I quit going to her as the few hours of pain relief didn't seem to be worth the severe pain of the treatment, especially when the beneficial effects only lasted a few hours.

My second PT was a man who was very empathetic, as almost all of the therapists I have met have been, and he only had me do very light stretching exercises. Then he would give me a massage and send me home with instructions to do the same exercises at home two-to-three times a day with five repetitions of each of about six different stretches. Of course being gung-ho, I asked if it would help if I did ten reps per exercise and he said yes. So that's what I did. My other appointments with this and the other PT had always been in the mornings when my pain is normally at its lowest. My third appointment with this PT was late in the afternoon—I hadn't taken my afternoon medication, and my pain was always worse in the afternoon. When I got there I just started bawling and had to leave and didn't go back.

The next PT I was referred to was more of the same. Each different doctor, my regular primary care physician, and my pain-management doctor sent me to their favorite PTs. The first one was recommended to me by two of my own patients. This last PT said he didn't know what, if anything, he could do for me that hadn't already been tried. I appreciated his honesty and went to him a few times—very light stretching exercises—and then I quit going to him as it didn't seem to be making any difference.

Then I started going to aquatherapy and it seemed to be helping, although the only thing I did was walk back and forth in the heated pool, sometimes raising my knees up high, and sometimes stretching my legs out to the side or backwards while holding on to the side of the pool. I went from only being able to walk for about five minutes before beginning to hurt, to over an hour at my last session. After one of the longer sessions when I walked out of the steps leading from the pool, I was amazed at how heavy I felt from just the walking out of the water (my weight had been being supported by the water) to the full gravity out of the water. The heated pool is amazingly soothing.

The aquatherapist was taking it very slowly with me. My first session with her was at her office, not in the pool. She, like the others, took my history and then had me stand up and bend backwards and then forwards. It was in the morning and I hadn't taken a pain pill yet that day. After bending forward, when I stood back up I was in severe pain and had another meltdown—just sobbing for a few minutes. I asked her for some water and took one of the pain pills I had learned to always have with me. It was not pleasant for her or me. It's embarrassing for a grown man to cry and sob, and embarrassing for someone to watch a grown man cry uncontrollably. So after that she was quick to ask me how I was doing, and if I were hurting we would stop for that day.

Going to all these therapies and dealing with my pain was taking up a great deal of my time. And my pain was getting worse. Sometime in July 2008, my daughter accompanied me to Honolulu on Oahu to meet with two different pain specialists, one recommended by my primary care physician and one by my pain-management specialist. My daughter had to go with me because the combination of my pain and the side effects of the various pain medications I was taking would leave me confused and they—my extended family—and I were afraid I'd get lost and not make the appointments. I'm glad she went with me, though I hated to admit that I needed the help.

We went over from the Big Island to Oahu the night before the appointments and spent the night. We got there early enough to go to see an art exhibit called "The Bodies." It was beautiful. Someone had taken the various parts of the body—skeletal system, lungs, heart and blood vessels, nerves and the brain, and many other parts—from real bodies, and preserved and mounted them for display. I would have loved to have taken some pictures but that wasn't allowed. I've since learned that these "bodies" may have been taken from prisoners who were killed for that purpose.

So why is this part of my story? Well, I could walk and ride a bike and not hurt but standing looking at exhibits leaves me in excruciating pain after only a short time. Shortly after we entered the exhibit, I told my daughter that I couldn't go on; I had to find a seat. There were several people in white, doctor-type coats there to explain and answer questions. Fortunately, one of them saw me sitting and must have seen the pain on my face as she asked me if I needed anything. I said, "Yes, I'm in pain.

Do you have a wheelchair I could use?" They quickly got one for me and with my daughter's help I was able to see the exhibit. I did feel a little guilty riding in a wheelchair and then at the end getting out of the chair and walking away. A person looking on couldn't tell that I needed the wheelchair.

The next day we went to the consultations with the specialists; one in the morning and one in the afternoon. They both had copies of my MRIs, X-rays, and CT scans. They interviewed me and had me do some bending and stretching. They both said that there was nothing that they could suggest that hadn't already been tried and that I should take my medicine and learn to live with the pain. The only hope that they could give me was that maybe it would gradually get better. They likened it to a football player's injury to a muscle that sometimes would take a year or two to heal. I was not happy. My pain wasn't getting better; it was getting worse.

My primary care physician at home started me on *Oxycontin* rather than the hydrocodone I had been taking up to four times a day, and I could take the hydrocodone for breakout pain. That is pain that, for whatever reason, gets worse and breaks through the shield of the regular pain medication. At first I was overwhelmed by the medications. They left me groggy and wanting to sleep all the time but gradually, as my body got used to the medications, I was able to function adequately. At that time I was also taking *Lyrica* and *Neuronton* at varying doses, and laxatives for the constipation that comes with narcotic medication.

Several months prior to my pain becoming so bad, I had scheduled myself to go to the "Maui Writers' Conference." It was to be held in Honolulu from August 27, 2008 to September 1, 2008. I had some real fears that I wouldn't be able to make it and even thought of canceling my reservations. Then I had the thought of asking my daughter to accompany me to the conference and since she is a writer too, she agreed. I packed up all my medications and off we went. In general it was a great conference, except that I ended up crying profusely during two of my 10-minute consultations—these are the best part of the conference when prospective writers get a chance to pitch their book to potential agents—and I wasn't able to complete them. Who wants to represent a writer who can't even do a 10-minute presentation without falling apart?

I was still taking heavy-duty pain medications and due to the pain and meds, I was unable to attend any of the evening presentations. However, one good thing did come out of the conference. I went to a presentation about writing a self-help book. I came away from that seminar with the idea to write this book. From my point of view, anyone who struggles with surviving chronic, severe pain is a true hero.

In late September or October of 2008, I got another referral, this time to a neurologist. He saw all my prior records and did some nerve tests and said that I was extremely hyper-reactive and diagnosed me as having "poly-peripheral neuropathy", or in English, a loss of feeling in both my feet and my right hand and arm. I agreed with him about my feet as they often feel numb, hot, and tingly. I didn't agree with his tests, which indicated I had nerve damage in my right hand and forearm, as I didn't have any symptoms in those areas at that time. He didn't prescribe any treatment so I stopped going to him. My other doctors, while acknowledging that I had some peripheral dysplasia—pain and loss of feeling in my feet—discounted it as non-significant, as I could still feel a cool alcohol swipe on my feet and legs. With each doctor or therapist I had to again and again tell them that my pain didn't radiate down my legs and I wasn't diabetic or anything similar.

In October 2008, I had a visit from my friend who lives on the mainland. She had extolled how wonderful her doctor was at the Cleveland Clinic. My friend gave me her doctor's name and various means of contacting him and I asked my pain doctor if he would send all my information to this person who was a DO, Doctor of Osteopathy, not a medical doctor. Osteopathy is a system of medicine based on the theory that many diseases are caused by misalignments of bones, ligaments, and muscles, and that correcting these through manipulation can cure the problems.

The two doctors consulted over the phone—my MD had sent my records to the DO—and they agreed that there wasn't anything that the DO could suggest in the way of diagnostic or treatment efforts that hadn't already been tried, except for seeing a DO. The DO in Cleveland gave my pain MD the names of some DOs on Oahu—I live on the Big Island—which would mean another plane ride to get there.

My pain doctor knew a DO who worked in Waimea—the northern part of the Big Island. So rather than spend money for another plane trip for my daughter and myself, I made an appointment, early in November 2008, with her. My daughter drove me to the appointment as I was in pain and had to take pain pills—and I often don't remember what the various doctors tell me. The DO wasn't really interested much in the medications I took, or rather she asked me about some of them but not all. Then she put me on a massage-type table and manipulated my legs and hips and then gave me a massage and told me that she wouldn't work with me if I didn't have a "back program." She gave me a handout with stick figure drawings on it of five different, very simple, leg, and lower back exercises to do. After 45 minutes she said we had to quit as she had other patients to see. On the way out we stopped at her receptionist to make a follow-up appointment and found out that she didn't take any insurance and the bill was $275.00. I was somewhat stunned. Later, I did get $71 reimbursed to me from my insurance company.

My daughter was very impressed with this DO because she was the only one who gave me some specific exercises to do and insisted that I do them or she wouldn't treat me. I was very unimpressed for a variety of reasons, the most important of which to me was that I found her to be very un-empathetic and cold; I just didn't like her. It was as though she didn't really understand chronic, severe pain. And in fact, other doctors and therapists had given me exercises to do and vitamins and minerals to take.

As I almost always tell my patients, one of the most important criteria they need to use when choosing a psychologist is whether or not they made a connection with the therapist and felt good about the first session. I didn't, so when I got back to Hilo I canceled my follow-up appointment with the DO.

I have, however, continued to do the simple exercises she gave me both morning and evening religiously. I don't know if they are doing any good, but they aren't hurting me, and all of the doctors tell me I need to do things to exercise and increase the strength in my back. She had also suggested that I stop riding my stationary bike and start walking, as she felt that sitting on the bike was putting too much pressure on my coccyx—the lowest extremity of the spine. I have started walking but haven't given up riding my bike, as other MDs suggest I continue both.

By mid to late November 2008 my body's tolerance to *Oxycontin* had built to the point that it wasn't effective in relieving my pain. This was to be expected and it happens with almost all pain-relief medications. At this point I was seeing my pain-management doctor almost weekly and he tried me on another type of pain medication, *Kadian*, but for me it wasn't effective. He then started me on *Fentanyl* transdermal patches, 50 mcg. These are placed on the skin and are supposed to last three days. They have the advantage of allowing the medication to be absorbed through the skin and thus are less damaging to the liver. After about a week of these I said I had to have something else or a stronger dosage. What I was taking wasn't working for me. However, the doctor didn't want to try a stronger dosage, as he was afraid of severe problems if I were to miss a dose. He did arrange to get permission from my medical insurance company to try using two 25 mcg patches that I could alternate and change every day so that at any one time I had 50 mcg a day but was replacing the oldest one with a new one each day. This worked well for me, and the pain was manageable.

I'm amazed at what small things can cause me a severe setback. I was at my pain doctor's office for a follow-up visit and was telling him how well I was doing and how proud I was of myself for having been able to cut my break-out pain pills from four a day to one a day. He wanted me to bend over to check out my flexibility again. I told him I could do it but that it would hurt me. He said to go ahead and like a dummy I said okay, bent over, and was screaming in pain. For the next two weeks my break-out pain medication use was back up to four a day.

Sometime around the first part of December 2008 I got approval from my insurance company to get a TENS unit. TENS stands for "transcutaneous electrical neural stimulation." It is a battery-operated unit about the size of a package of cigarettes with four wire-insulated leads that go to "patches" that you stick on your skin in an X pattern directly over the pain area. Then by turning two knobs on the unit you can change the frequency and intensity of the stimulation. This really worked for me. It causes a feeling like buzzing or fingernails scratching extremely rapidly over the pain area. The doctors don't know how it really works, but the theory is that the electrical stimulation interrupts the pain signals to the brain, thus eliminating the perception of the pain, if not the source of the pain. It's similar to what happens to a patient who has tinnitus—a ringing in the ears—when they play music through their headphones, the tinnitus goes away. The pain doesn't go away, but the TENS unit and/or music mask the pain signals from going to the conscious brain.

There are problems with the TENS unit though, especially if wearing the patches over the lower back. They are very hard to put on by yourself if you live alone as I do. The patches are supposed to stick to the skin and have an eighth of an inch of sticky gel that covers the patch—each patch is about one and a half inches square—and sticks to the skin as well as provides some insulation between the bare patch and the skin. Unfortunately, when they are on the lower back and one is sitting and moving, at all, the patches get pulled and pushed against the fabric of whatever you're sitting on, and wearing, and eventually they get pulled off the back, and/or the electrical wires get pulled from the patch.

This results in a rather comical process—at least for other people watching—of repeatedly receiving, intermittently, a mild to moderately painful shock. This first happened to me when I was initially trying out the patches and went out to supper with my son and daughter and proudly showed them the TENS unit clipped to the waist of my pants. After about an hour or so sitting in the restaurant, I started jumping like a puppet on a string, saying "Ouch, ouch", as I frantically reached for the knobs to turn the unit off.

The medical supply house, which supplied the unit, told me that the four patches that came with the unit would last a year. What a joke; they didn't last a day with normal activity. When

I went back to get more they were surprised at my problems and reluctantly sold me four more at $18.00. I asked if they didn't have some that would stay on better and they said that they only had the one kind. Calling around to other medical supply stores on the Island didn't result in my finding any better patches. Fortunately for me, one of my patients had a very large supply of them and gave me some of hers. I've tried various ways of trying to put them on with various types of adhesive tape and bandages over them to hold them on. It's quite a process to get them on, and then taped on, and I look like I've been severely wounded with all the tape all over my lower back.

When I went to the medical supply house to get the TENS unit, I looked around at all the various medical supplies and equipment they had on display. I asked the salesman if they had anything else for low back pain. He pointed to a cushion that was on a chair and told me to sit on the chair and lean back into the cushion. When I did that the cushion began to buzz and gradually began to heat up. It felt really good and I said I'd take one of those. He fitted it to my car seat and plugged it into my car's cigarette lighter.

I asked if he had anything else. He said, "Boy have I got something for you," almost like a used-car salesman. It was a curved board about 24 inches long by 16 inches wide, made of hard plastic, and had a gentle curve from high at one end to low at the other—like the shape of the spine. It had two rows of knobby posts with a channel so that the rows of nubs fit on either side of the spine and the posts could stick up into the trigger points on the spine. He had me try it on their showroom floor—no one else was in the store—and I found it painful, as he said I would. He encouraged me to breathe through the pain and to relax. After about three or four minutes, I couldn't take it anymore and rolled off to my side and got up with the salesman's help. My pain, which had been at a 2 or 3 on the 1-10 scale, was gone. I bought the board called *TrueBack*. You can find it on the Internet by googling *TrueBack*. The pain relief lasted several hours and I started using the board for 15 to 20 minutes morning and night. It was after I started using this device that I really started to get better and to use less pain medication. If I had to pick the most effective elements in my treatment of pain I would say that for pain-symptom relief, pain medication is best, along with the TENS unit. For treatment of the cause of my pain, I would say it was the *TrueBack* and stretching and exercise.

The first part of December 2008 was a difficult time. I woke, not only in pain, but the whole process left me exhausted, even after nine hours of sleep. I was back to not wanting to live, I was just too tired, all I wanted to do was to go back to bed and sleep. But I wrote more of this self-help, rode my stationary bike, and then went to see my granddaughter in a Christmas play. I have to exercise to keep from gaining more weight and I know I feel better afterwards. My stepson called as I was just starting to write this and just hearing his kind and enthusiastic voice picked up my spirits. I was still extremely tired but wanted to live to hear his stories. He has a way of talking that makes life humorous, and now I feel better. Such simple things affect the perception of pain.

Some two or three weeks after my last entry in the above paragraph, I felt like I may be getting a bit better, knock on wood. I had avoided one of the traps of the pain-medication cycle. It was time for my appointment with my pain-management doctor and in the past I had terrorized myself with worry about what I would do if he took away my *Fentanyl* patches. They had just begun to work and I had been successful in reducing my medication use.

So I had kept the fear at bay and my doctor agreed that I was doing well and we could continue with my current medication regime. Then he wanted to check my flexibility and he again asked me to bend forward towards my toes as far as I could. I told him I could but that it would cause me severe pain as it had the last time. I don't think he believed me, and like a fool, I bent down as far as I could (about 12 inches from the floor) and started screaming in pain. Some of his staff members came to see if everything was okay. I was back up and was okay, but for the next eight days I was back to using higher doses of medication. I swore to myself that the next time he, or anyone else, asked me to bend over to check my flexibility I wasn't going to do it. Shit. I knew I shouldn't have done that and I won't again. It's like asking a person to stick their hand in boiling oil to see if it still hurts.

My life still revolved around my pain and all the things I did to try to manage the pain. In a typical week I'd have three to four doctors and/or therapy appointments. Every day I had to monitor my pain-medication intake—did I take that pill this morning or not? I'm physically unable to do most of the things I took for granted, like bending down to pick up a piece of paper, or fixing my ice maker, or kayaking out to my son's boat. I remember to put on a new *Fentanyl* patch at night. On any given day there was a small window of opportunity when I could function for two to three hours. At these times I was able to write and/or do my digital painting. I still see patients but I am limited to two half days a week, from 11 AM to 3 PM. I've had to quit my 4 and 5 PM appointments as the pain was too bad. I'm in pain when I see my patients and often have to stand and pace, or rock from foot to foot in my office. But my patients seem to understand, as most of them are chronic-pain patients too. I seem to have begun to specialize in this area.

On weekends and on days when I'm not seeing patients I just want to sleep and avoid the pain, but I get up and do my back exercises and then all the activities necessary for daily living like grocery shopping, washing dishes, cleaning up, returning mail and phone calls, etc.

In January of 2009, I was still in pain but still doing better. I walked and/or rode my bike three to four times a week, still took my pain medications as prescribed, and did my back exercises. I could begin to see some future and have some hope that I would continue to get better. I knew I still had to face getting off the *Fentanyl* patches. During the last year of my life I had been so limited by my pain that I couldn't, and didn't even want to think of the future. My goal was to continue getting better by doing everything that I could and not doing things that might set me back. I also wanted to have this self-help book finished by the time the Maui Writers' Conference was to take place in September 2009.

Through January 2009, I continued to do better. I had been able to cut down on my *Fentanyl* patch use and was continuing with aquatherapy. My TENS unit helped tremendously. I could see some hope. Even if I never got much better than I was then, I could see living with this, where I couldn't six months ago. I had started walking and was getting into it but developed severe pain in the metatarsal pads on both feet, that at least for some time had made me quit walking. I saw an orthopod—one more doctor—about the pain in my feet. The ups and downs of my "progress" continue. I've been able to reverse the trend of gaining weight and have even lost a few pounds, which I find encouraging. I got off the antidepressant medication with no ill effects on my mood.

I'm at the end of the first draft of this book and will put it down now for six weeks and then re-read and edit it. I hope to have it ready for publication by fall of 2009.

Now, March 4th of 2009, my journey continues and next week I'll edit the first draft. I continue to improve and have reached the point where I can say to myself that if it never gets any better than this I can live with this pain as long as I have my coping tools. My pain medication has been further reduced and I continue with my therapies, as listed in the paragraphs above. I've even reached the point that I can see or believe that at some time in the future I may even be free of the tyranny of this pain, which has so hobbled my life.

It's now July 2009 and my pain has gone down and up. Currently way down. I was doing so much better that I bought a new kayak and started reducing my pain meds and was still doing well. But then *!#** happened again. I had gotten over-confident. I think it must have been one kayak trip that was too long, along with a continued reduction in my pain meds. Over the last three weeks it has gone back to being almost as bad as it ever was. I can't even call it living, sleep is all messed up, and then when I do sleep that is all I want to do. With so much pain and lack of energy I'm not able to even go for a walk, or ride my bike, or kayak. It's been a bad four weeks.

I had another MRI done last week and will call my pain MD today. I had to get off of the *Fentanyl* patches as I had developed a bad skin rash from them. The new meds—morphine sulfate ER—aren't working, and I barely have the ability to do anything. I can still see patients but I have to take many more pain pills and often have to stand and rock from leg to leg during therapy sessions. I was struggling, barely holding on.

In two months it will be time for the Hawaii Writers' Group to meet again on Oahu. Maybe I'll find an agent to publish this book but at this point my pain says I don't care. I just hope that my pain level isn't as great as it was at the last workshop.

I had just gotten in my latest edition of AARP July/Aug 09, and on the front cover was printed in bold yellow, "Stop Back Pain Now: New Therapies That Could Change Your Life", by Perry Garginkel. WOW! My eyes lit up and I got all excited. Maybe this is it? Not. The author notes that up to 85% of all Americans will have some form of severe back pain in their lives and most of that is chronic. He did get one thing right: "Part of the frustrations in treating low back pain—both for the physician and for the sufferer—is that outcomes vary so dramatically from one patient to the next.

[That's what I've been trying to say.] Although acupuncture might offer relief to one person, it may do nothing for another." Unfortunately his "new information" was just a rehash of stuff I already knew. Hopes dashed on the rotten rocks of despair.

The only thing I got out of the article was an old Zen saying, "Before enlightenment, chop wood, carry water; after enlightenment, chop wood, carry water." It means that no matter how much you may know about the cause of the pain you still have to deal with the symptoms.

My last few weeks towards the end of July have been filled mostly with much more severe pain and suffering. I know how to handle it better but it still ain't easy.

During the first part of August 2009 I made another dumb mistake—how many times do I have to keep doing this before I learn? My pain meds worked okay, but they left me exhausted. I needed to replace some curtain hooks on the curtain in my office. All it took was a step stool and some new hooks: "I can replace them myself. I've done it several times in the past; I can do this . . . not." And now my back hurts worse. You'd think I'd have learned by now. "Oh when will it end? When?"

The last few weeks of August 2009 have been really bad again. My back seems to be getting worse and the pain medication makes me too sleepy. I got the results back from my latest MRI and they showed some mild degenerative disk disorder or bulging in disks L4 and L5. My pain-management MD gave me the option of doing a "diskogram" procedure, which would be very painful but might be able to pinpoint the area of damage. Then if they can find the specific area causing the pain he suggested I might consider going to Texas where there is a world-class MD who is doing experimental trials of "fibrin sealant injections" into the discs. Before I do anything like that, I'd do a lot more research on my own so that I'd know what that involves. The MD—who my pain MD recommended—is supposed to be the best in the world and they are in Phase III of their clinical trials of this experimental procedure and have had "very good" results. I would want to know a lot more about that before I proceed down that road.

I told my pain MD that I wanted to wait for a few weeks. I had just started some new chiropractic treatment two times a week. A friend and colleague had said this person was really good and that I should give her a try. I thought, "Why not, I've tried so many things; this one might help." My state of pain at that time and medication stupor was so bad that I had to cancel going to the Writers' Conference even though the fees are non-refundable. Bummer, but I feel that it would be a waste of time and beyond my ability to do in my current state of pain. Fing #%&@**.

But then Hope raises its head again. I had seen a new chiropractor—middle of September 2009—who did a really through job of evaluating exactly where the pain was and which muscles were weak. At the last session she said she felt she had found the base cause of my pain, which was due to the back abdominal muscles on the L4, L5 discs being "mushy" and very weak on my right side. She gave me a very specific and simple exercise of lying on the floor and bicycling my right leg while holding my abdominal muscles as tight as I could, keeping my back pressed completely flat to the floor. I could definitely feel the difference between the right and left leg when I did this exercise. EURIKA—after a week of doing these exercises I was doing much better with very low pain levels, but the acid test would come when I tried to get off the morphine meds I was taking. I REALLY HOPED THIS WOULD WORK, because I was not looking forward to the next option of a diskogram. She saw me for five sessions and I was ready to quit, adding her as another of the long list of experts I've seen.

It's now the middle of October 2009 and I'm still in severe pain. I do the exercises faithfully and they do help some, but not enough, and I'm trying to cut back on my pain meds. But it doesn't seem to be working. I can barely keep the tears from flowing as I try to talk to my patients.

July 15, 2010. A lot has happened since my last entry to this book/journal (almost 13 months). I'm still in severe pain, which has gone up and down for several months. I had a friend come to visit and she had to go home early as I was in too much pain.

I don't remember when it was but I had been feeling so good that I got myself a new kayak. It has bicycle peddles attached to a shaft that went through the center of the hull to penguin-type flippers under the keel. Since I didn't have to use my hands to paddle I could go fishing. I also had a friend who I would go kayaking with. Unfortunately, the last time we went out (which must have been several months ago) we stayed out for 4 or 5 hours. I didn't feel any pain at any time while paddling, but when we got back to shore I literally couldn't straighten out and get out of my kayak. My friend had to pull me out with his hands. I still didn't hurt—I had good lumbar back support and was enjoying my life. BUT, from that day to the present I haven't been back in my kayak. I've continued seeing my various MDs, but primarily Dr. Ruhland on a monthly basis, and trying a variety of different medications. I'm currently on *Oxycontin* 20 mg and *Dilaudid* 2 mg, 3 times a day, *Savella* 50 mg in the evening, and a variety of different anti-depressants and sleeping medications. I still take hydrocodone about 2 or 3 times a day for break-out pain.

I feel like I'm back to square one—which is common for chronic-pain patients—and am, again, not wanting to live. I've had to cut my hours of my clinical practice from 11 AM to 5 PM two days a week to 12 PM to 4 PM two days a week, and my pain severely limits my ability to do much of anything. I just want to lie in bed on a heating pad all day.

All this time I'd been forcing myself to exercise daily by walking, but mostly by riding my stationary bike. All my MDs want me to lose weight so I have been riding more. I've lost about 25 pounds, as everyone says it will help me and my back if I lose weight.

I don't know how it dawned on me and why the MDs didn't pick it up, but IT

FINALLY HIT ME. IT WAS THAT VERY ACT, BENDNG OVER MY COMPUTER, THAT ORIGINALLY CAUSED MY PAIN, AND HERE I WAS RE-INJURING MYSELF ON AN ALMOST DAILY BASIS LEANING OVER RIDING MY BIKE. Neither I, nor any of the "professionals" made the connection that it was the very act of bending over that was re-injuring my back. Just sitting straight up in my kayak was enough to kill me (later) with pain and the same was true for bending over and riding my bike. My stepson did suggest I quit doing everything and then gradually add things back to my daily routine to see if I could identify what was continuing to cause my pain. One osteopath suggested I walk more and not ride my bike as it put too much pressure on my coccyx, but she didn't get it that it wasn't the sitting but the bending over that caused the pain.

Currently my MD is thinking of sending me to Seattle to see some specialist there. I will hold out for three months to see if my hypothesis is correct and my back will get better if I no longer continue bending over to ride my bike. I'm gaining weight back but will settle that later. I hope that by the time this book gets published, I'll be mostly pain free. I didn't make my date of getting it published by this year's Writers' Group Convention, but the convention was canceled for this year due to the recession.

It's now the first part of August 2010, and in agreement with my pain-management MD I've started the process of getting off opiates. I had been telling myself that I wasn't addicted, as I didn't want the drugs for the sake of the drugs but for the pain in my back. I now know that I am/was addicted to the opiate drugs. Two nights ago I didn't take my nightly dosage—per agreement with my pain MD—and it was a really bad night, cold sweats and shakes, but they had given me medication to help with these, *Clonidine*, and I took a *Valium* too, but it was still a very hard night. Last night was my second night with no evening dosage, and again a hard night. All I can do is lie in bed and suffer—I take my morning dosage of 20 mg of *Oxycontin* and 2 mg of *Dilaudid* and have cut my mid-day meds to 10 mg of *Oxycontin* and 2 mg of *Dilaudid* and no evening dose. I certainly have new respect for drug addiction and how hard it is to get off them. Yes, I've had to admit that I was a drug addict, medically prescribed, but still a drug addict. Once I get off of them I hope I never have to go back on them ever.

My pain MD talked to his colleague/friend in Seattle who said that he couldn't see anything to do that hadn't already been done, so it looks like I won't be taking any trips to the mainland for more consultations. I am scheduled to receive some more back injections that work for about two weeks in taking away the pain. I hate this dependence and really realize how hard it is for drug addicts to get off the addiction. Tears rolling down my face, I try to take my mind off of it by talking to friends on the phone and watching mindless TV. Hopefully, by the time I'm to start aquatherapy again, I'll be off all the opiate meds. Can't write any more now.

August 14, 2010. Feel like I may as well be dead; though I can still see a light at the end of the tunnel. I'm now on a single daily dose of 1, 20 mg *Oxycontin* and 1, 2 mg *Dilaudid*, which I try to take at about 11AM daily. Have to force myself to do anything but lie in bed. I now have a stair stepper that keeps me upright and I've succeeded in turning the weight trend around so that I'm again losing weight. But some days I have to force myself to use it.

August 21, 2010. Now down to one 10 mg *Oxycontin* a day and haven't taken one today, just one hydrocodone 7.5 tab. My back is not hurting too much and the worst of the withdrawals seems to be gone. I did have another set of facet injections from my pain MD this last Thursday, and as expected was worse the next day but better now. Keeping on living—or trying to.

August 26, 2010. Now on my sixth day of no *Oxycontin* or *Dilaudid*; I just take 1 to 2 hydrocodones a day. Withdrawal from the heavy-duty narcotics has been rough: night sweats, nausea, and no energy. As I've said I have a new understanding and respect for addicts who get off the drugs. However, given the choice of severe pain and no addiction, or managed pain and addiction, I'd take the addiction. I've only been able to get off the hard drugs because I'm in less pain since I quit riding my bike. When I'm doing therapy I still have to stand up frequently and rock back and forth, and am still limited to four appointments on Tuesday and four on Wednesday.

August 31, 2010. Now over the worst of the withdrawals and back in aquatherapy; and again am beginning to see a light at the end of the tunnel. I'm not going to push it though. I've written to every publisher in the writers' market re: self-help, but either get a rejection or nothing. My current goal is to be able to get back in my kayak in the ocean by January 2011. I'm off of almost all narcotic meds. I do take a hydrocodone on average once every 3 or 4 days.

I can much more clearly see the connection I knew intellectually existed between the stress/anger and more intense pain. The stair stepper wasn't working right and it took numerous calls and threats on my part to finally get someone to come out and give me a new one that worked correctly. I hadn't made myself that angry in 30 years and my self-induced anger went straight to my pain in my back. I teach people how to handle stress and anger; I should be able to manage better than this!

9/2/10 and I'm now completely off all narcotics; I'm still in pain but it is manageable. I'm doing aquatherapy in a heated pool, and I take some muscle relaxants. If by Feb of 2011, I haven't gotten an agent or publisher I will do self-publishing so that I will have a book I can give to my pain patients and say "Read this. It might have some good information about how you can decrease your suffering and manage you pain more effectively."

It is now the 16th of June 2011 and I'm finally going to send this final version to my publishers, iUnivers, and hope to have it available for sale by the end of July 2011.

I did have another break through, again from one of my patients. We were talking about our various back pains and how we were coping with them. I had told him that the only time I wasn't in pain was when I was lying down on my bed with a rolled towel under my lumbar region. He suggested, "Doc, why don't you come over here and lie on the couch and I'll sit in your chair." I then told him that he could try the recliner instead of the couch. And I pointed out that if I pushed my laptop computer out of the way, that the chair I was sitting in and was also a recliner. I then showed him by pushing the computer (that was sitting on a metal arm that swung out from a low table I had it attached to) and pulling the footrest lever up and pushing back so that I was in a reclining position. Boom, it hit me. If I could find a way to be reclined and still have access to my computer to take occasional notes of what we did in the therapy session, then I wouldn't be in any pain and would not have to stand up and stretch every 20 minutes.

Within a week I had found an "Air Desk" that met my needs perfectly and for the last two days that I have seen patients, I put my feet up on a footstool and tilt my chair back, and bingo, I was not in pain and the Air Desk gave me easy access to my computer.

Don't get me wrong. I'm still in pain, but it is at low levels, say a 1 or 2 on a 1 to 10 scale. I still can't sit in a chair at anyplace for more than 20 minutes without having to stand up or the pain would go quickly to a 6.

But overall I'm doing much better than I was in handling my journey with pain. It is still a slow process and I still occasionally do something to aggravate my back and then my pain level goes up again. But now I have hope and best of all a life. I can write and paint all using an air desk while I'm on my bed.

Chapter 8:
Prior Experience with Pain Patients

I've been a clinical psychologist for over 38 years and over the last few years have started seeing more and more severe, chronic-pain patients—mostly 'Workman's Compensation' cases. My job as a psychologist member of the informal pain-management team is to help the patient address the psychological issues that are always and inextricably associated with severe, chronic pain.

The first step in psychological treatment is to deal with the stigma—still present, though not as bad as it was 30 years ago—of seeing a psychologist. Most pain patients initially perceive the idea of a referral to a psychologist as a slap in the face. It's like the patients are thinking, "I'm not crazy. I'm in pain. What do I need to see a shrink for? You think I'm making this up?" (Bumper sticker: Shrink hemorrhoids not people.)

"Of course you're not crazy," I tell them, but if they try to tell me that their pain doesn't affect them emotionally, then I tell them that they either aren't being honest with me or with themselves. You'd have to be crazy not to be depressed and/or upset emotionally at the pain and subsequent loss of function.

Once we get past that hurdle we can move on to some of the coping strategies I talk about later in this book. I thought that I was fairly compassionate and empathetic in dealing with these patients, but until I had my own chronic, severe pain, and drug addiction, I couldn't really—at a gut level—relate to how traumatic it is. It's like a psychologist trying to tell parents how to raise their children when the psychologist has never had any children (I have three, all grown). Even now I can't say "I know how you feel." That's another slap in the face. No one knows how you experience your pain, how you hurt, but I now have some deeper understanding and even more empathy. I can feel their pain experience because I have some of the same experiences with my chronic, severe pain and the same frustrations of trying to get treatment that works.

Ironically, it is often my own patients who suggest things that they have tried that I end up suggesting to my own pain-management doctor and using in my own life. One of my patients asked me how I could spend hours a day helping others when I was in so much pain. My reply was, and is, that helping them to try to have a life larger than their pain helps me to have a life larger than my pain.

I find that I now use the analogy of chronic pain for all of my patients even if the issues for which they are seeking help are not expressed in any physical pain. Any of the life-altering events that would bring a person to see a psychologist are like chronic, physical pain. The problem takes over the patient's life and they must find some ways of coping with it, of having a life larger than the pain or problem in their life, whatever those problems are.

PART TWO

Chapter 9:
Impact of the Problem

On the Patient

Chronic, severe pain affects **every** aspect of my life from sleep, to sex, to living, and to the right to the pursuit of happiness. It makes me more grouchy and less of a person. One time at a pharmacy when I was trying to get a pain prescription refilled and they had said it was too early to get a refill, I got very angry with the pharmacist when she said, "I know how you feel."

"No you don't. You can't unless you've had severe pain," I hissed at her.

She said, "I've given birth to three children; I know what pain is."

"You're right," I said, "but even that pain is not the same as chronic pain that doesn't go away." I walked off in a huff.

I later went back to apologize to the lady for snapping at her when it was really my pain talking, but that is no excuse.

And sex. Forget it. I used to have a fairly active sex life, even if alone. But now, due to the pain and the side effects of the various pain and anti-depressant medications, I seldom even have the urge, and when I do, I often can't ejaculate. Orgasms are a great release of hormones and relieve the pain—at least for a while, if you can have one.

Chronic pain negatively affects **every** aspect of one's life—you become less social and have a tendency to isolation and severely reduced social interactions. You don't want to talk to people for fear that they will ask how you are and you don't want to tell them, "I f***ing hurt. Leave me alone." Or worse, you don't want their unsolicited, if well-intended, advice. "Well, have you tried . . ." Yet the social isolation leads to more depressed feelings and thoughts of uselessness and hopelessness—and yes, sometimes self-pity. There are the persistent thoughts of not wanting to live this way; and at times wanting to die.

Then there is the expense of the drugs and the various other forms of treatment, and all the time spent going to doctors and other health practitioners. Having chronic pain is a full-time job. I don't know how poor people handle it. They get some help from welfare but that whole process is demeaning and depressing in itself.

It takes me two hours to get up and get going each day with various exercises, pill-taking, putting on TENS patches, etc. I don't sleep well, often waking in pain. Sometimes I'm able to roll over and go back to sleep, and other times I have to take another pain pill. Nighttime has become a dread. Will I be able to get to sleep? I try to turn out the light between 10 and 11 PM, but often it is 1 or 2 AM before I get to sleep, and of course that messes up my whole schedule for the next day.

I've tried almost all the types of sleep medications and all of them lose their effectiveness over time; or rather, my body builds up a tolerance to them. I've tried extra-hard firm mattresses to the nova-foam type, which is very soft and molds to my body. For me, I find that the latter is best. I use body pillows. You name it; I've tried it.

I think the worst personal impact is the huge loss of function—so many of the things that I used to do and take for granted I can't do now. Forget getting on the floor for any reason, whether playing with kids or trying to untangle computer wires. I have two grabber-type things—one in my bedroom and one in my kitchen—so that I can squeeze the handle of the top of the stick and the pincher on the other end will then pick up the object on the floor. I can't go out after 5 PM or so, unless I have someone to drive me, as my pain gets too bad at that time of day and I have to take pain medications, which makes me unable to drive and generally poor company.

Taking all the narcotic mediation makes me feel like a "druggie." I take one medication and it doesn't work for me so the doctor prescribes another. Then the pharmacy doesn't want to fill it as they tell me I already have a prescription for another medication that does the same thing. I then need to explain that I'm no longer taking that prior medication. As one pharmacist said, "Does your doctor know you're taking this?" I felt like saying, "No stupid. You caught me. I stole his Rx pad and forged his signature."

"Of course he does. He's the one who prescribed it," I say in frustration.

Then another big put down. My insurance company made me sign a "drug contract", as though I were taking drugs for pleasure or because I was addicted to them. I know, intellectually, that there are valid reasons for requiring things like a drug contract. Still, it contributes to feelings of being treated like a "druggie", or a criminal, or a second-class citizen.

While all of these negative impacts are there and often overwhelming, there are some positive aspects or consequences of the pain, as evidenced by my earlier reference to Senator McCain. My job as a psychologist—and for myself as a chronic-pain patient—is to get the patient to find some meaning and purpose beyond, or larger than, their pain. The victories in doing this are in very small increments, inch-by-inch and minute-by-minute, hour-by-hour, and day-by-day; to shift the focus from what I/you can't do to what I/you can do.

Pain forces—it doesn't allow any options—one to slow down. And then if you're willing, it allows you to take pleasure in the very simple things in life. Like the Bobby McFerrin songs, "Don't Worry, Be Happy" and "Simple Pleasures Are the Best." That's easy to say but oh so hard to do. Live in the present. Taste the coffee, feel the sun and wind, see the clouds, listen to the music, enjoy a hot shower. The past is gone; the future is yet to be;

and right now—while you are reading this—or me, as I was typing it—is the only time we are alive, right now, this moment in time. Enough of that bull-hockey sophistry—a plausible but misleading argument. It's misleading in that the pain demands attention NOW. Take a deep breath, exhale slowly, and tell yourself to relax. Maybe you'll be able to find some small pleasure for that day.

My pain has made me a much better therapist and person, I think, but then I am biased. It has made me write this book and to be much more appreciative of every minute of life with all the people with whom I interact. There are no meaningless, thoughtless interactions, they all are vastly important.

Effects on Others

While the impact of pain on the patient is very debilitating, except for the actual pain, it can be equally debilitating for those who love and care for the pain patient. They begin to feel hopeless and powerless too. They hate to see their friend, spouse, child, or parent in pain and not be able to do anything about it. For a person who lives with the pain patient it is even worse because they are constantly aware of your pain.

They watch you take medications that they know are highly addictive and have negative side effects. They have to pick up the load of doing the work that you used to do. They go through the stages of pain also.

Denial: "There's nothing wrong with your back. Just quit complaining."

Anger: "Why do I have to do all the work around here? I'm f***ing tired of hearing about your pain. You know I have pain too."

Depression: "I feel so bad. I can't help you. I don't seem to have any interest in life anymore either."

Bartering: "If you can just pull your act together while I do this one job, I'll make it up to you."

Acceptance: "I guess we'll just have to get used to it. This is the way our life is going to be. And while it's not what we thought it would be, we can make some good moments."

Of course some spouses can't stand the pressure of your pain and suffering—especially if you don't choose to focus as much as you can on the simple things that you can do—and they choose to leave the relationship. They may leave literally by divorce or just by moving physically and mentally away. Or they may move away by staying at work or being in a relationship with someone else. They may turn to addictions of gambling, drugs—stealing your drugs—alcohol or pornography, or others. No doubt chronic, severe pain puts a huge stress on the relationship and if the marriage was already unstable, this may be the straw that breaks the camel's back.

It is hugely important that all parties have open and supportive communication. Of course feelings get hurt about the pain, whether you're the one with the pain or the person living with them. Both patient and caregiver need to be able to talk about their feelings and needs and work on compromises that work for both. They need to focus not on the limitations caused by the pain, but rather on what you both **can** do in your lives together. Many people really want to help you and you have to be able to let them, while maintaining your own boundaries and dignity. Some caregivers want to take over completely and a sick, symbiotic relationship develops where the pain patient stays helpless and more dependent on the caregiver than necessary, and the caregiver won't let the patient do even the things they can do for themselves.

People who used to be friends don't know what to do or how to deal with you so they start to stay away from you, or they become overly solicitous and constantly offer unasked advice about what you should do. If you have the type of pain that doesn't have a readily visible source, like the loss of an arm, or leg, or a disfigured face, some may look at you with scorn, as if there is nothing wrong with you.

Some physicians have a very hard time dealing with chronic-pain patients because they don't know what to do with them or how to ease their pain and suffering. Some doctors actually begin to resent the patient's demands on their time. If they can't fix it with surgery and/or medication, they are often at a loss as to what to do. Patients have often told me that their surgeon or other MD has told them that there is nothing that they can do for them—that the patient just has to learn to live with the pain. These doctors don't have enough sense to tell them how to do that, i.e. live with the pain, nor do they have the sense to refer them to someone who might be able to help them to learn how. That is why it is probably better to see a pain specialist (with a team of helpers) rather than a general or family practitioner.

As a psychologist, I remember seeing my first chronic-pain patient years ago and listening to their long litany of complaints and failed treatments. I too wondered what I could offer them and didn't look forward to seeing them. Over time I began to realize that they are like other patients and need someone to listen to them—that in itself is a huge part of therapy—someone who will listen and isn't expected to make it better. I gradually began to build more and more coping strategies that I could offer my patients if they wanted them. Now, I actually enjoy seeing my chronic-pain patients, as we have deep and real dialogue about their lives and mine. Much of what I have learned, in terms of helping chronic-pain patients, has come from other patients.

At work, bosses and/or supervisors don't know how to respond to a person with chronic pain who is trying to regain some job functioning. They expect them to recover too quickly and often push them. The patient goes along with this as they want to return to full capacity and they push themselves to the point where they are re-injured. When professional athletes are injured it may take one or two years or more to recover, but there are very few employers who will give an injured worker that long.

Chapter 10:
Treatment

The Treatment Journey Begins

Your journey may begin with a specific car accident, a specific work or home injury, or it may be the cumulative effect of a repetitive-motion injury such as carpel tunnel syndrome, or cashier's elbow, or from surgery or an illness. In my experience, most people are so worried about getting back to work or about losing their jobs that they go back to work too soon, and either re-injure themselves or exacerbate their injury. Back to denial. "I can go back to work; it only hurts a little bit. No pain no gain. I've been injured before and it didn't keep me from work. Besides, I've got bills to pay."

Now the injury is even worse. In my case, my injury was caused—as best as I can figure it out—by bending over my computer for hours at a time, writing my first novel. The muscles and ligaments in my back got so stretched out of shape that now they won't relax.

So now let's talk about the things that happen on the journey of pain.

Please remember that each person's journey is unique to that person and what works for one may not work for others. Also, again, I strongly recommend that you consult with your own physician before trying any of the coping strategies listed below.

The System

The health-care system, at least where I live, in Hilo, Hawaii, is broken almost beyond repair, and I suspect that is the case in most rural communities and inner cities in America, if not the world. Or maybe it's just broken for those who don't have the money for the best care.

I'll limit my comments to my own neck of the woods. Here, doctors are chronically over-burdened. Many people who have good health insurance can't find a physician who will take them on as a patient. Many doctors leave the area as they can make two-to-three times as much money in other metropolitan areas. Even when a person finds an MD who will accept them as a patient, if specialty care is needed, one has to first get insurance permission and then often they have to go to Honolulu on Oahu—the place where most people think of when they think of Hawaii. What most people don't realize is that Oahu is a different island and you must take a plane to get there from Hilo. There are no ferries.

There are answers to these problems, but that is a political essay and I'm not going there.

The most egregious—conspicuously offensive—breakdown, however, is in the "Workman's Compensation" system. In this State almost all companies are required by law to carry Workman's Compensation insurance for their employees. Workman's Compensation is so bad that there are very few doctors who will agree to see a Workman's Compensation patient. Why? Because any treatment for the patient must be approved in advance by the Workman's Compensation insurance carrier. This approval usually takes several months, if not years before the insurance company will authorize the treatment.

"Well," you might say, "couldn't the injured worker use their regular health insurance?" No. Not unless they lie—which is fraudulent—because if they tell the truth that the injury happened on the job, then the doctor must report it as such, and then their regular medical insurance won't pay as the insurance company says—correctly—it's a Workman's Compensation bill.

The State law in Hawaii says that if a treatment plan is sent to the Workman's Compensation insurance carrier and the carrier hasn't denied it in writing within 7 to 10 days—I'm not sure of the exact time but that is not the point—then the treatment is automatically approved. However, the reality is that if the doctor provides the treatment without written authorization, they may never get paid. I know. I've had that happen to me. And if it is authorized you'd better get it in writing. Again, I know from my personal experience and from hearing other doctors tell me of Workman's Compensation non-payment. I've had verbal authorization for treatment. The primary care physician who is referring the patient to me assures me that they have verbal authorization and almost begs me to go ahead and schedule an appointment to see the patient. Unfortunately, when I send my bill in for payment the Workman's Compensation carrier denies it, saying that the treatment was never authorized. As is said about medical charts: "If it ain't written down in the chart, it never happened." If you don't have the authorization in writing, it didn't happen.

This isn't an isolated incident. It's rampant and one of the reasons most doctors won't take a Workman's Compensation patient. Even if the authorization is in writing, Workman's Compensation carriers often still refuse to pay. So what can the doctor do? I can't abandon the patient just because Workman's Compensation won't pay. That is unethical. I didn't go into the healing profession to make money. I did it to help people and so I go on and continue seeing the patient anyway, paid or not. Many doctors avoid this problem by not accepting Workman's Compensation patients to begin with. Once I've accepted them into treatment, I've made a commitment to them that isn't going to end if Workman's Compensation decides, after two years or any other time, to discontinue any further treatment.

Even if the treatment is authorized by the Workman's Compensation carrier, payment is often delayed for months or years. Doctors and other health professionals can't stay in business and not get paid, hence the reluctance to accept Workman's Compensation patients.

The Workman's Compensation carriers deny treatment and/or payment for treatment for years and save millions of dollars.

The "adjusters" are the persons assigned by the insurance carrier to manage the Workman's Compensation case. Some are actually very helpful. Others seem to be evil incarnate. They say they are "here to help you"—the patient—when in fact they do anything they can to block and deny any treatment and/or payment. They act as though it is their own personal money that is to be spent on the Workman's Compensation patient's treatment. I wouldn't be surprised at all to find out that they are paid a bonus based on the number of denials and delayed payments they manage to accumulate. The insurance carriers make billions of dollars from the Workman's Compensation premium fees charged to companies. Part of these fees is taken out of each worker's paycheck.

It is a very sad state of affairs, if not downright criminal, the way these Workman's Compensation cases are treated, but the system is set up so that by law it can't be sued. Workman's Compensation is supposed to be there to help an injured worker get well and/or retrained so that they can return to some kind of gainful employment or if they can't return to work due to their injury, to pay them compensation based on the amount of income they could have made if they hadn't been injured. In my experience this never happens. I don't know why. Are the insurance companies so stupid that they don't comprehend the economics of the process? Do they really think that they are saving money by not paying for treatment for the injured worker? Don't they understand that if they provided timely treatment that they would be likely to be much more successful in getting the worker back to work? It is not unusual for a Workman's Compensation case to go on for 10 or more years, and when a settlement offer is made to the injured worker, it is for a very, very small fraction of what the worker could have made if they hadn't been injured.

Maybe there is some economic logic that favors the insurance carriers by denying and delaying treatment. Some workers become so worn out by all the delays that they give up and settle for a pittance—say 15 to 25 thousand dollars. How long can you live on that if you're injured and can't go back to work? Well, of course, there is "Social Security Disability" for workers who can't work due to their injury, but that system is going broke too. And again, try living on the small amount that SSI pays.

Maybe the insurance companies have it right. They are in business to make money not to help injured workers. So maybe they do understand the economics of what they are doing, and that is evil.

However, they have no understanding of the urgency of medical need for treatment. Treatment delayed is often treatment denied. If the injured worker had gotten the right kind of treatment within the first few months of injury they might have been able to return to work. The lack of timely treatment often exacerbates both the physical pathology causing the pain, as well as the emotional trauma to the patient. It usually takes about two years before a patient is successfully referred to me for psychological treatment. That delay is not only the fault of the insurance company but is sometimes due to the lack of knowledge of the physicians and reluctance of the patients to see a psychologist because of the stigma that is still attached to seeing a shrink.

In a typical case, a worker is injured—a fall, explosion, or other accident at work resulting in physical damage to legs, back, neck, and/or the brain to name a few. The injured worker is sent to his or her regular primary care physician, or to the ER, or an Urgent Care Center—and treated with minimal use of resources and sent back to work, perhaps on light duty. Here, both the physicians and/or the patients may be partly responsible. Physicians are under pressure to not use expensive diagnostic resources unless really needed and the patient may say something like, "I'm okay Doc. It just hurts a little and I need to get back to work." Denial at work again.

If the worker doesn't have a regular medical doctor he/she must then try to find one who will take a Workman's Compensation patient, and the cycle begins.

One patient I treated was so nice and polite—this was his very nature—that when his doctor would ask, "How are doing today?" the patient would reply with a smile, "Okay, I'm alright," when in fact he was in severe pain. It took some convincing to get him to be more honest and tell the doctor how much he hurt. If the patient isn't honest with the doctor, the doctor doesn't have any way of knowing how much pain they are in.

After this initial treatment, the doctor may make referrals for more diagnostic tests such as CAT scans, blood analysis, MRIs, X-rays, and others. It typically takes six months to a year to get authorization from the insurance carrier. If the patient finds that they are in too much pain to continue working, then the trauma of the Workman's Compensation process begins.

This typically involves numerous referrals and waiting for authorizations. Other experts and consultants may become involved. Patients often become frustrated with the system and on advice of friends and other workers, who have been through the "system", they may hire an attorney.

Patients may be sent to vocational rehabilitation, to various other forms of therapy, some of which may help and some of which may cause more harm. If they are lucky and/or knowledgeable they will get sent to a pain-management (PM) specialist. Most PM doctors use at least an informal team approach to treatment that usually involves a variety of helping disciplines, including psychologists.

Eventually the patient will be sent—by the insurance company—to an MD or Ph.D for an independent medical examination (IME), which is supposed to be what the name implies, an independent, i.e. someone who is fair and unbiased, not on the insurance company's side or on the patient's side—but rather neutral. This person is to evaluate the medical evidence in this case, to determine if the patient's physical problems, pain, and emotional distress were caused by the worker's injury or due to some pre-existing condition. Whether the patient is malingering, exaggerating, and making it all up is assessed. The IME is also supposed to evaluate the current and past treatment and make recommendations for further treatment and/or return to work. The evaluation usually takes place in one day and involves a face-to-face interview that may last 30 to 60 minutes and then three to five hours of paper and pencil psychological tests, such as the MMPI-2 (a widely used personality test) and a review of any medical records of prior treatments and/or evaluations. For patients from Hilo this means either an early morning flight—6 AM—or the night before and then a late evening flight back to Hilo.

I'm not sure you have the picture yet. These IMEs usually don't take place until well after the pain from the injury has become chronic and severe. The IMEs are anything but independent and unbiased. To begin with they are paid by the Workman's Compensation insurance companies; I've been told they get between $10,000 and $20,000 for each evaluation depending on the number of pages. Most of the reports consist of page after page of quotes from other doctor's reports. Whether consciously or unconsciously, the IMEs are influenced to say what the insurance companies want them to say—e.g. the patient's injury was pre-existing. Or they are malingering, because if they don't say what the insurance companies want them to say then the insurance companies will quit making referrals to them. The Workman's Compensation insurance companies then use these IME reports to justify denying any further treatment.

Other evidence of the IMEs being biased is statistical in nature. If 99% of the patients referred to a doctor for an IME are found, by that doctor, to be malingering and/or that the injury was due to some pre-existing condition, then that is blatant evidence of bias. If 100 work-injured patients were referred for an IME, probability theory would indicate that at least half of them would be found to have injuries that were due to the work injury. So if a particular doctor finds that 99 of the 100 Workman's Compensation patients referred were malingering and/or that their injuries were due to a pre-existing condition, then that would be de facto evidence that that doctor is biased against the Workman's Compensation patients referred to him or her.

That would be like a judge, who is supposed to be fair and unbiased, who found 99% of the cases involving a black defendant guilty while only finding 1% of similar cases involving white defendants guilty. That is outrageous, and so are the IMEs.

In fairness, this same statistical argument could be made against me as for 100% of the Workman's Compensation patients I see, I find that their pain is causally related to their work injury. Some 25% of the time I find that they may have had a pre-existing condition that was exacerbated by the work injury. But the patients who are faking it don't come to see me, whereas all the Workman's Compensation cases get sent for IMEs.

Here is more evidence of bias. One IME MD actually wrote in his report that, "Mr. X, like all chronic-pain patients, is exaggerating his symptoms . . ." Talk about bias, he has prejudged all chronic-pain patients without even seeing them. I'm sure that not all IMEs are biased but almost all of the reports I have seen—somewhere between 150 and 200—have been against the patient. Curiously, if the patient pays for his or her own IME it is often found in the patient's favor. In my practice I have only seen two IMEs that were favorable to the patient and one of those partially retracted his statements after he was contacted by the Workman's Compensation carrier and questioned about his report.

Again in the interest of full disclosure, I, too, am paid by the Workman's Compensation insurance carrier for treating the patients. There are three major differences between myself and the IME doctors. One, I'm paid a lot less, $144.22 per treatment session. Two, I continue to receive referrals, not from the Workman's Compensation carriers but from MDs who are the primary care physician, even though I write my disagreements with the IMEs in my treatment notes. Three, I base my conclusions on 10 to 60 or more treatment sessions, as well as interviews with spouses, other treating doctors, and reviews of records, whereas the IME relies on one 30 to 60 minute interview (often much less time than that), a review of the records, and paper and pencil psychological tests that are not valid for predicting malingering or any pre-existing condition for any specific patient. And even if there were a pre-existing condition, it could be exacerbated by the work injury.

To sum it up the plain truth is that the insurance companies' primary purpose is to make money—my primary purpose and the primary purpose of the treating doctors is to help the patient get better.

Many Workman's Compensation patients develop what I call the "Workman's Compensation syndrome." The process goes on so long they become depressed both by their pain and loss of function and the way they are treated, or rather denied treatment, by the Workman's Compensation system. They become fearful to the point of paranoia, thinking that the system is out to get them. One patient even thought—even though he knew it was irrational—that the Workman's Compensation carrier was going to burn his house down to destroy his records. Some patients report feeling that someone is watching them. They become fearful of going out in public for fear someone will take a picture of them smiling or someone will report that they were seen laughing and that this will be used as evidence against them. One patient actually had his picture taken while he was looking into the hood of his son's car and the Workman's Compensation carrier tried to use that as evidence that he wasn't injured but was malingering. In fact, in that incidence I had prescribed to the patient that he help his son with his car as that was one of the activities he had enjoyed prior to his injury. He wasn't doing any of the work, but had looked in the hood of his son's car and made some suggestions to his son about what he thought might work in fixing the car. The Workman's Compensation carrier backed down.

Nonetheless, most Workman's Compensation patients develop this irrational fear that if they are seen laughing or even going out shopping, that someone will report them and the Workman's Compensation carrier will try to use that against them. So they become even more depressed and withdrawn. Chronic-pain, Workman's Compensation injured patients can laugh and go shopping and do many things and that doesn't mean that they are malingering or that they aren't in pain, or that they can work full or even part time. I even write prescriptions for them to laugh and to go out to the extent that they can but to not overdo it.

I thank whatever Gods there may be that I'm not a Workman's Compensation patient. If I were I'm sure some IME would say that I'm malingering as none of the initial physical evidence showed anything wrong with my back, yet I have severe, chronic pain. Unfortunately, the state of medical science is not refined enough to locate the source of pain for many patients. One small nerve that can't even be seen, except under a high-power microscope, can cause a severe toothache and the same is true for nerves in the back and other parts of the body.

Chapter 11:
The Doctors

Almost all doctors go into the healing professions to help others. Unfortunately, there aren't enough and they are overwhelmed by the demand and the need to see a large volume of patients in order to pay their staffs and to make a living for themselves and their families. Many of them do make a lot of money but they spend 12 or more years making nothing and piling up huge student loans before they begin making good money. Most of their salaries are not anywhere near the obscene levels of professional athletes, movie stars, or CEOs of the large insurance companies. Maybe we should go to socialized medicine like Canada, but I don't think so. What we need are more physicians despite the studies that show that when more MDs are produced, medical costs actually go up. Yet medical costs are not going up anywhere near as fast as educational costs. There are many lawyers—and we need them despite all the jokes about that profession—and legal fees are reasonable and attorneys are reasonably available.

Even if you get to see a doctor, they are not the all-knowing gods that they are trained to think they are. In today's medical world the patient needs to be an active participant in their own treatment and not just blindly do what the "Doc says." Those days are over. To get effective treatment now, you—the patient or the patient's family—have to take an active role in educating yourself about your symptoms and diseases and treatments. Sometimes you need to educate your own physician about your condition and the good doctors welcome your participation in your treatment. It takes some of the burden off of them.

For chronic pain it's important to write down your symptoms and track their frequency and circumstance, when they are worse or better, and share that information succinctly with your doctor in written form. Trace your medications, minerals and vitamins, exercise, activities, and pain levels. Have your questions written down so you won't forget them and you will stay on track. In my case I've had to have my former wife or daughter or girlfriend go with me to appointments as, due to my pain and the pain medications, I don't remember what the doctor said. The only way your doctor can really help you is if you give him/her full and honest information about your symptoms.

Some doctors are good and some aren't. In rural areas it is hard to shop around but it can be done. Don't give up. Don't be afraid to quit seeing the one you don't like or the ones who you don't think are helping you. They can't make the pain go away, in most instances, but they do have a large arsenal of things that they can do. However, the most important member of your treatment team is **you**. What you bring to the treatment in terms of motivation to get better and to take responsibility for what you can do is critical. There is one commercial for a national health-insurance company that I think typifies the outmoded thinking of the past. The commercial shows a canoe being paddled on a lake and the voiceover says something to the effect that the patient is one of the paddlers and the MD is the steersman who guides the canoe over the rough waters of medical care. The analogy is outdated. Most MDs don't have time to be the steersman, that's your job. The MD isn't even one of the paddlers, they are knowledgeable consultants—and are critically necessary individuals—who can make suggestions about where you need to steer the canoe and may even be able to do operations and prescribe medications that will help.

The doctor or doctors aren't going to make you well or better, you have to do that. They may make suggestions, prescribe medications, do surgeries that help or they may make suggestions that will take you in the wrong direction.

Chapter 12:
Other Therapists

There are many "other" types of therapists or helping professionals: doctors of osteopathy (DOs), physiatrists (MDs who specialize in physical medicine and physical therapy—how this is different than an MD I don't know), physical therapists (PTs), occupational therapists (OTs), acupuncturists, massage therapists (MTs), aqua therapists, mood therapists, dietitians, faith healers, herbalists, naturalists, pain-management teams/clinics, pain support groups, marriage and family therapists (MFTs), and chiropractors to name a few. I'm sure I've left some out. They each have their own acronyms and language. Some help some people and not others. You have to find what works for you and if it isn't working and/ or you're not learning how to cope better or at least maintain an adequate level of functioning, it may be time for you to try someone else.

It's my job—and yours, if you're in pain—to find the ones that are right for you—not an easy task, in fact a very daunting one. I've tried most of them. Some of them work, to some degree, but some made my pain worse. Unfortunately it's all trial and error. Even the ones who made my pain worse were all very nice to me—it wasn't that they were mean, it was and is that my pain is so overpowering, like a vengeful God that demands almost constant attention, even devotion, that their suggestions/treatments at that time didn't work for me.

As an example, Harvey comes under the heading of "other healers" of no particular school or training. All of my friends ask me how I'm doing and often ask me if I've tried this or that for treatment. It is usually more of a pain to listen to their well-meaning suggestions than it is a help. A psychologist friend of mine suggested a guy named Harvey who she and her husband both went to for back problems. You had to make an appointment three months in advance to even get to see him. He wasn't taking any new patients at the time but her husband had an appointment in mid-January 2009 and I could have that appointment if I wanted it. At that time it was late November

2008 and I said yes. They didn't even know his last name until they looked it up but they highly recommended him. He only took cash and it was $55 for a 20-minute session. By then I was ready to try pretty much anything and since I respected my friend's opinion, I accepted. When I asked Harvey if he had any degrees or credentials he said no, that he learned how to do his treatment by doing things with patients. But surprisingly, therapists like him serve a large number of people very effectively.

When the time for the appointment rolled around I was doing a bit better. The appointment was at 11 AM, so my back was just beginning the daily decline into stronger pain. Harvey's office was in a small strip mall. I went in not expecting much. He, like the acupuncturist I had described before, didn't have me fill out any paperwork and only asked extremely minimal historical information, and that was while he was working on my back on a massage table. He did some massaging and said that I was very tense and that one leg was shorter than the other—one of the PTs had said the same thing—and then he did some things that I would expect a chiropractor to do. He snapped my neck left and right and then had me hold my hands behind my head while sitting up, elbows together, and then he got me in a body hug from behind and "snapped" my back. He did that two or three times and said that was it and asked me how I felt. I said fine and then I started to hurt again and he again "snapped" my back and I felt better, though I didn't expect it to last.

He told me to call him and he would "work me in" if I was in any more pain and scheduled me for another appointment in February 2009. I went back for another treatment session with him but discontinued after that, as I felt it wasn't helping me.

My Patients

My patients are the unsung heroes of my treatment and of their lives. Some of the best treatment suggestions I have gotten have come from other chronic-pain patients who I see professionally as their psychologist. One of the most important things other patients can offer is Hope. If that person can go on, then so can I. They have been able to help me find sources for TENS patches and have suggested a wide variety of medications, some of which I have tried and all of which I discussed with my pain MD.

Friends and Relatives

Chronic pain affects not just the person but the whole family. Patients who have supportive family members and/or friends are very fortunate. They serve as drivers to take you to appointments and do many other caregiving things like foot massages and getting you out of the house, being quiet when you need to be quiet, and listening when you need to talk.

The Experts

The experts may be experts as certified by their various professional organizations, but that doesn't necessarily mean that they know what they are doing or that they will be of any help to you. You are the only real expert on you and your pain. You won't get the help you need if you sit back passively and wait for the experts to fix your problem. Experts are often so narrowly focused that they forget that they are dealing with a whole person. They become blinded by your pain and don't see a bigger picture of the person's life. And there are some "experts" who are a total waste of time and money. As someone once said, "An expert is someone who has a briefcase and is 500 miles from home."

I've consulted several experts and haven't found that they were any more help than my local pain-management MD. In my case they all say that I need to take my pain medications and learn to live with the pain. Only one of the so-called experts even said anything about how to do that, i.e. live with the pain.

Learning how to do that is the journey that I have taken and that you must take by trial and error, and by using some of the coping strategies I discuss below. Sometimes "experts" are downright dangerous. I have one patient who received serious brain injuries in a work accident. After several weeks in the hospital and head scars so deep you could put your fist in his head, he was left with diminished motor functioning and ability to talk. An "expert" neuropsychologist from the mainland said this patient had to be faking it because he did worse on some of her tests than known brain-injured patients. Of course he did worse. Did this expert even look at his crushed skull? He did worse than most known brain-injured patients because he is worse. Her conclusions were based on 15 minutes of testing and the overly long latency of his verbal responses. I've seen him professionally for over 60 sessions and interviewed his wife during most sessions. He is brain injured. He's not faking it. He can't do any better.

As a clinical psychologist I'm aware of these so-called binomial choice tests, which compare a person's response to known brain-injured patients' responses, and to those who were known malingers or fakers. What this expert and others often forget is that their "test" data doesn't take into account this specific individual's responses and his history, and the data of his actual functioning over time. It's too technical to go into in depth and this is not a technical book, so enough of that.

Chapter 13:
Medications

Medications. Wow, wouldn't it be great if there were a magic pill that would stop the pain and let you live your life the way you used to? Unfortunately, no such pill or combination of pills exist. There are too many pain medications for me to go into any depth on them. In sharing my journey earlier in this book, I've shared many of the medications I've tried.

With medication there is always the question of weighing the benefits versus the costs of taking the medication. Not just dollar costs—though those have to be considered too—but side-effect costs, which include possible addiction. Some people are allergic to many of the narcotics and/or may become habituated to them so that they need to keep taking higher and higher doses in order to get the same treatment effects. On the positive side, the research that I'm aware of indicates that it is less likely that a person who is taking the pain medication for pain will become addicted than a person who takes the same medications for recreational and/or emotional use. I would also make the argument that if my choice is to be addicted or in severe pain, I would choose addiction.

Other side effects of medication can be just as serious. To name just a few of these we can include: impotence, inability to ejaculate, loss of sexual desire, constipation, irritability, memory impairment, cognitive confusion, sleep disturbance—not sleeping or sleeping too much—loss of energy, weight gain, and many others. I've experienced all of these. Then it is not just the pain that keeps you from doing the things you used to be able to do, but the pain medications also. But again, one has to weigh these side effects versus being in severe, debilitating pain. Is it worse to be debilitated by the pain or by the side effects of the medications?

When I'm past a certain level of pain-medication use—on any given day—I know that I can't drive and have to depend on someone else to drive me wherever I need to go. The effects on my cognitive abilities are such that I have to have someone go with me to my doctors' appointments to help me, because I don't remember what happens.

My personal choice is to use the medications, and it has been, and is, a trial and error process of finding which medications work for me. I also use other coping strategies as much as possible to decrease my dependence on pain pills.

Chapter 14:
Coping

If you haven't gotten the message by now, coping is what this book is all about: how to cope with the insidious, constant, overwhelming, severe pain. The shotgun approach that I describe below has some problems. When you try a lot of different things at once or at the same time, you won't know which one was effective in helping you. But it hurts too much to take an academic or research approach of trying one thing at a time to see if it is effective. Usually it's not just one thing, but a combination of things, medications, and the things discussed below that are effective.

Shotgun: Kill First, Ask Questions Later

I tell my patients that their task or mission (and mine), should they choose to accept it, is to develop their very own pleasure menu, like when going into a restaurant and opening the menu I have several options to choose from for my coping pleasure. I had to, and you have to shift the focus from what you could do, but can't now, to what you can do now. In Hawaii there is a saying, "If can, can; if no can, no can." I had to develop my capacity to enjoy the simple pleasures of life that I could do. I still get upset at the things I can't do, but I try not to dwell on it.

The strategies or coping methods listed below are not in any order of importance. Some of them may seem very simplistic but they do work. Try them or not and use the ones that work for you, modifying them to fit your particular needs. All of these are done usually in conjunction with traditional medication and are not meant to replace medication and/or other types of treatment.

Psychologist

"We shall never know ourselves until we have taken a long look back along the rocky road which brought us where we are" (Mary Renault).

This is my part. I love what I do. I've been doing it for 38 plus years. Psychotherapy, to me, is one of the deepest relationships a person can have with another human being. Patients tell me their deepest, most secret thoughts, because I am a stranger—at least when we first start—bound by ethical rules of confidentiality, and they want to tell someone who will listen. That is really one of the most important parts of therapy, listening, not making it right or fixing it, just listening. We all want to be listened to and as we go through our lives, most of the time no one is really listening, not our friends, lovers, colleagues, and certainly not the many clerks in the stores we frequent. Very few people really listen; they are all thinking of what they want to say and/or something else entirely. At best we sometimes get an implied social contract with friends, that if I listen to your story then you'll listen to mine.

For chronic, severe-pain patients it is even worse. People get tired very quickly of hearing about your pain. Even the pain patients get tired of hearing themselves talk about it. Enough already; get a life. But that's just it. I can't. Don't you understand—the pain is my life. I guess that's why I can and do listen as though it is a new story each time with each patient, because it is. I do understand. That is one thing that my pain has given me, a deeper ability to listen and to understand other people's pain, whether physical, or emotional, or both, as it always is both. I express it in my paintings and now in this book, and in my continuing therapy with my patients.

Many MDs and psychologists don't want to treat chronic-pain patients partly because they don't want to listen to their pain and because they don't know what to do to help the patients who don't get better. So many times my patients tell me how much they appreciate just being able to talk to me and feel like I understand them. I tell them how much I appreciate them. Some come for weekly sessions and some come once a month. We talk story, and share parts of our lives. There is minimal bullshit.

You may be able to handle your problems or issues on your own and not need the expense of a psychologist. The same is true for weight training, playing any sport, learning any skill from speaking a foreign language to playing a musical instrument, doing legal or accounting projects, to building a house, but it sure is easier to have a professional coach/teacher to help you on the journey.

A good psychologist, however, is not just a good listener—bartenders and hairdressers do that (well some do)—but also someone with knowledge and experience in human behavior about why we do the things we do and how we can change. He or she is like a coach or an emotional personal trainer.

Time for another joke. How many psychologists does it take to change a light bulb? Only one, because we are smart. However, there is a catch—the light bulb has to really, really want to change. It's funnier in person.

I suggest some simple criteria in selecting your psychologist. Do you feel like you made a connection with him/her? Do you feel like you were listened to? Do you want to go back? Are they helping you learn and/or practice ways of coping with your pain, to have a life larger than the pain, to the extent that you can?

With my patients—when we get to the part about coping, and that is after the listening—I suggest all kinds of strategies for them to consider and/or modify for their own use.

An 11-year study at Ohio University's Department of Psychology, published in the December 2008 issue of *Cancer*, the peer-reviewed journal of the American Cancer Society, showed that if women with breast cancer received a quality psychological intervention program, conducted by an experienced therapist, they improved their survival rate from death from cancer by 50%. And they had a reduced risk of death from all causes, not just cancer. There were 227 women in the study and 114 received the added psychological treatment and 113 didn't.

The authors attributed the results to a reduction in stress. It couldn't have been the stress that they reduced but rather the way the individual women **responded** to the stress. The psychological interventions " . . . included strategies to reduce stress, enhance their relationships with friends and family, coping effectively, improving mood, [and] altering health behavior . . ."

That's some strong evidence. If they can do that for cancer patients, I hypothesize that there are similar health benefits for chronic-pain patients.

You may have noticed that I don't have a section on psychiatrists. Psychiatrists are trained primarily in physical medicine, and psychologists are trained in human behavior and thinking and feeling and how to change behavior through ways other than medication. Psychiatrists are good for what they are trained in and that is medicine and medication. Most of them don't have the time or training to do psychotherapy. They are in too much demand to do medication checks.

So let's get on with it. To the coping strategies.

Again, please remember that not all of these will work with all patients and I again, strongly advise you to consult with your physician before trying anything I suggest.

Breathing

Breathe. In Hawaiian, Aloha means sharing the breath of life with you. Breathing is the single most effective and simplest skill for coping with stress. I'm talking about taking a deep breath in through your nose—fill your chest and belly with air—hold it a few seconds and then exhale "slooowly" through your mouth and drop your shoulders and tell yourself to "relaaaax." I've been told that there is a scientific reason for breathing in through the nose and that is because there are small follicles in the nose that extract nitrogen from the air (nitrogen is the stuff laughing gas, nitrous oxide, is made from). I don't know how true that is but it sounds good. Personally, I do the breathing in and out through my nose; just my personal preference. Modify it to fit your style.

Do this deep slow breathing 10 to 15 times an hour. It is physically impossible for your body to be both tense and relaxed at the same time. If you breathe deeply you will oxygenate the lungs and blood system and relax. I'm constantly telling my patients about the need to breathe. The osteopath I went to see told me I needed to breathe more. She was right.

What does this have to do with pain management? Let me describe the vicious cycle of pain again. When you are in pain, the pain causes your body to become tense, and the more tension you have the worse the pain is. So anything you can do to decrease the tension in your body will reduce your pain. Unfortunately, one of the reasons people abuse alcohol and drugs is to relax. "Relax, we'll have a few drinks, have a few laughs . . .": the line from the first "Die Hard" movie.

Breathing only does so much but it is critically important. For acute pain especially, you'll often hear people telling you to breathe through the pain. You do the same with both the acute and chronic stages of pain.

Relaxation

Relaxation is a skill that you must learn and practice. Pain makes tension, which makes the pain worse. The "fight or flight" response is the body's natural, inborn—you don't have to learn it—response to danger. It has survival value. If there is a perception of danger, your very survival depends on your ability to fight or run away from the danger. While that may have been fine for cave men, it's not very effective in the modern world. Most of the dangers we face on a daily basis can't be solved by fighting or running away. In fact the biggest source of stress—the danger signals you perceive—is from your own mind. Your mind gets your body tense to fight battles that may never occur. This is a normal biological process. While it is a normal process, it becomes pathological if you remain in a constant state of fight or flight arousal.

Relaxation is not a normal process in modern society. We even fight battles in our dreams. Relaxation most often must be learned, and like any skill, it takes time and practice to do it well. It's true that some people are naturally relaxed and go through life very calmly, never getting upset by much of anything. Most of us aren't like that.

So how do we learn this skill? It starts with the breathing I described above. After learning how to breathe, I teach my patients two basic types of relaxation; one is muscle relaxation and the other cognitive relaxation. Muscle relaxation is a process of tensing and then relaxing the major muscle groups of the body—hands, biceps, triceps, chest, back, stomach, thighs, calves, toes, forehead, eyes, neck, and jaw, etc. If you remember some of your basic biology, you know that the muscles that control the movements of these body parts are called "striated" muscles. If you tense the muscles, then when you relax them, they will relax to a greater degree than they were before you tensed them.

Tense—as tightly as you can without causing pain—both of your fists for about five or ten seconds and then relax them. Try it now. Put the book down and try it.

Did you notice the difference? That state that you feel after you release your fists is muscle relaxation. If you had two hours to go to the gym to workout, you'd feel much more relaxed after a good workout. However, most of us don't have two hours a day to work out. The muscle relaxation I've described can be done in a few minutes.

Cognitive relaxation is just closing your eyes and imagining a relaxing scene. Like sitting in a very comfortable chair overlooking a clear, blue ocean, with a clear, blue sky and gentle, cool breeze, a very safe and secure place where no one can hurt you. Again, take a few minutes now and put the book down, close your eyes, breathe slowly and deeply, and try to picture in your mind's eye your own very peaceful and relaxing place.

Can you picture it? Can you feel yourself relaxing?

You can do both of these on your own but, especially for the cognitive relaxation, it helps to have a coach suggesting what to picture. The very act of telling yourself what to picture requires some thought, which causes some tension. It is much easier to do by just following directions from someone else. I give my patients a CD that has my voice giving directions on how to do both types of relaxation. Each is about 12 minutes in length. I stress repeatedly to my patients to not do any of my directions if it causes any pain.

Almost universally, my patients tell me that the CD helps them relax, which in turn reduces their pain. It doesn't last as long as a pain pill or tranquilizer, but there are no side effects, and you can do it as often as you need to, and there are no co-pay fees. They often use it as a sleeping aid, either to go to sleep or to go back to sleep if they wake up and have trouble going back to sleep. You can make you own tape or CD in your own voice using images tailored to your own needs and tastes.

The cognitive type of relaxation is similar to many types of meditation, and there are a wide variety of types of meditation. You have to try to find one that works for you.

Hypnosis

Hypnosis is all really self-hypnosis and/ or guided imagery and is very similar to the cognitive relaxation I described above. In addition, however, hypnosis can be used directly to address the pain. Many people who are very good subjects for hypnosis find that with training that they can learn how to control their pain much more effectively. Good subjects are people who have a very good and vivid imagination and are able to put aside their disbelief. Some can even learn to give themselves an imaginary injection of morphine and actually feel the same effects as if they had received a real injection. This also takes a great deal of motivation and practice. Don't feel bad if you aren't one of these people. It takes a very good subject and a skilled clinician to help guide a patient to this level.

If you want to try this, try to find a clinician who has experience using hypnosis in managing pain. I use this with some of my patients. One man I'm thinking of used an imaginary monkey on his back and he would take the monkey's arms off and throw him off but he'd keep coming back; he'd keep throwing him off and with some success was able to keep him off. Another patient pictured her pain as a huge elephant sitting on her chest and she pictured putting him on a diet and making him lose weight until he was almost completely gone.

Chapter 15:
Small Steps for Pain Management

Research has shown that test subjects can tolerate larger amounts of pain depending on the circumstances. In one study, subjects could leave their hand in icy cold water for longer periods of time if they focused on just the next breath or next minute rather than being told that they would have to keep their hand in the cold water for a specified amount of time.

While this is a simplistic strategy, and may not transfer from the lab to the real world very well, it may also be a useful tool, especially for the short "break-through" types of pain while you're waiting for the pain medication to kick in. Concentrate on making it through just one more breath and then one more, and then one more . . .

This is just another tool, which may or may not be useful to you.

Biofeedback

Biofeedback is a broad field of science that has to do with using feedback to the patient about their physiology in order to change their physiology. The most common types of biofeedback are the Galvanic skin response (GSR), the electrical conductivity—sweat—of the skin; thermal response (TR)—skin temperature; electro myogram (EMG)—the measurement of electrical response of the muscles; and electro encephalogram (EEG)—the measurement of electrical activity in the brain.

Biofeedback is a legitimate field of science and treatment. People who practice in this area are licensed and trained, usually as psychologists, in the use of these procedures to demonstrate to the patient that the patient can control all of these areas; sweating, temperature, muscle tension, and mental brain waves by conscious effort of the patient's thoughts. The devices used to do this are somewhat complicated but the basic principle is fairly simple. If the patient has a type of pain that is related to skin temperature, then the person is taught how to control their skin temperature. A patient's general anxiety level may be trained to be reduced by using the GSR. Muscle pains can be treated using the EMG, and the EEG can be used to train the patient in deep meditative states.

Although effective, it is not in wide use. I'm not sure why but it may have to do with the need for frequent training sessions, three to five times a week for several weeks that have to occur in the doctor's office. The machines are too expensive to let the patient take them home to practice with and it may not be covered by your health insurance. It also requires a highly motivated patient. But if it works for you it may be worth it.

I quit using biofeedback because of the reasons stated above. I used to use the GSR and EMG and temperature modes. It is effective, if for nothing else than to demonstrate, in a real way that can be scientifically measured, that the patient—with training and practice—can learn to control these bodily functions by their conscious thoughts. It stands to reason that if you are in pain it affects you physiologically—remember the "fight or flight" syndrome I discussed earlier. If you could be taught to reduce this physiological response, it could help you manage your pain.

If you're going to try this approach, I would suggest you find someone who is certified in this area and who has experience in using it for treating pain.

Doing/Trying

Some suffering appears to be necessary. It may be that the patient subconsciously wants to punish themselves for some perceived wrong. Many people have the egocentric thought that if something bad happened and they are in pain, it must be their fault. Maybe they did cause the accident or contribute to the accident and are therefore punishing themselves. They probably learned this pattern in childhood. If they are going to ever overcome this self-destructive tendency, they are first going to have to admit what they are doing or helping to do to themselves. This is best addressed in psychotherapy by a skilled therapist. In a weird way some patients even believe that they should suffer because they are making others in their life suffer due to their pain.

One therapist I worked with shared one of her tools she used with patients to get them to make changes. She had borrowed the concept from Alcoholics Anonymous. When a therapist suggests that a patient do something to cope with their pain, for example the old standby of taking a deep, slow breath, the patient might reply with something like, "I'll try to do that." Then to make her point she would ask them to try to pick up a pencil she had laid in front of them. When they picked up the pencil she'd say, "No, I didn't ask you to pick it up, I asked you to try to pick it up." The point she was emphasizing was to get them to see the difference between trying and doing. You either pick up the pencil or you don't. Although doing is good, sometimes the best you can do is to try and praise yourself for the effort.

Destructive Thinking

"Don't worry, be happy . . ." goes the song, " . . . cause when you frown you bring everybody down." Too true. It's easy to say, but oh so hard to do. It's like the patient says, "Don't tell me it doesn't do any good to worry. Everything I worry about never happens."

To worry is human nature. "How will I make the house/car/credit-card payment? What if this or that happens? What if it gets worse . . ."

on and on. If you have chronic, severe pain, you've got plenty to worry about from, "What if my medication runs out?" to, "How can I get to my next doctor's appointment?" It is normal and even beneficial to worry if it leads to productive planning. But it becomes abnormal and pathogenic—bad—when we obsess about our worries almost constantly, because this brings on anxiety and tension which (say it with me) makes the pain worse.

"So Doc, if it's normal and good, how do I keep from doing too much of it?" You learn to manage it. Like learning to manage the pain, or balance a checkbook. Use the Serenity Prayer. Or, set up a "worry time" and get a "worry journal" and then every day at your worry time you get out your worry journal. Then you **have to** worry and write down your worries over and over again until that day's worry time is over or until you're ready to let go of it for that day. At any other time of the day or night that you start to worry, you use thought stopping. Just say out loud "Stop it!" three or four times and then, if you must, you can write a quick note on a post-it to remind yourself to worry about that item when it is your worry time. If needed, you can use a negative, portable self-stimulator—a high-tech piece of psychological equipment, otherwise known as a rubber band. Put the rubber band on your wrist and pull it back a good distance and let it pop on the inside of your wrist—on the tender part. "That hurts Doc." Of course it does and that is to call your attention to what you are doing to yourself when you excessively worry or tell yourself bad things, like, "I'm a failure. It's no use. I can't do this." You're literally hurting yourself. If you want to hurt yourself go ahead and keep popping that rubber band and if one wrist gets too sore put it on your other wrist, and if it gets too sore put it on your ankle. SEE what you are doing to yourself. Feel the hurt.

These are just tools that you might be able to use to help you to not dwell so much on your worries. Don't confuse worrying with planning. Planning is good. Once a week you need to plan out the next week and month and year, so that you are organized. Organization and structure help reduce stress, which helps reduce pain. Plan when to see about getting new prescriptions so that you don't run out over a holiday or weekend. Plan for other things in your life. Then when you get up, you just follow the plan for the day and don't have to worry about what you're supposed to do that day. That is one of the ironies of being injured. It takes away the routine of work, so now you have all this time to worry and suffer.

When you were working you didn't have time to worry, you were too busy living and didn't have enough time to do fun things, and now that you have the time—due to the injury—you can't do them. Or maybe you can learn some new skills you didn't have time for before you were injured.

WHY is a question that is like worry. It is human nature to ask why. Why did this have to happen to me or now? If we just knew the answer to the question, "Why did this happen; what caused it?" then we would know how to fix it or deal with it. Maybe you can find an answer that will help you, for example, why is my back more sore right now? Well I just bent over to pick up something off the floor and I didn't squat with my knees but rather bent over from the waist. How many times do I have to do that to myself before I learn?

However, if you're asking the more generic question of WHY, you're probably wasting your time. There are thousands of answers that are provided in all the psychologies, philosophies, and religions of the world—it's God's plan, it's fate . . . If that works for you, fine. Most of the time, however, you might be better off asking, "How am I going to manage this? Why did I fall and hurt my back, or how am I going to manage my pain?" S*** happens. It's the nature of life. Clean it up as best you can.

Worrying and asking why are just two examples of how chronic, severe pain affects the patient. The repeated pain signals to the brain may cause what is called a "kindling effect" in that the neural pathways become so engraved in the brain that it takes less and less pain stimulus, as time goes on and the groves become deeper, to trigger the same severe reactions to what would have been, before the injury, a minor pain. To put it another way, the brain becomes so used to the pain signals that it now reacts to even minor pains as though they were major, severe pains.

"Life is what happens when you're busy making other plans" (source unknown).

I often give the following items to my patients to help them cope with worrying.

The Worry Game: A logical approach to control obsessive worrying

It was during World War II, around 1943. There were these two GIs (army soldiers—government-issued GIs) on the mainland waiting for orders to be shipped out to another base after they had finished basic training.

Some would go to other bases on the mainland and others would be sent to the War in Europe or the Pacific. One of the GIs (Moe) is talking to his buddy (Joe) who is very obsessively worried about getting shipped to the front lines in the war.

Moe says, "Hey, you got nothing to worry about; you either get sent overseas or not, right?"
Joe says, "Right."
Moe says, "Well if you don't get sent overseas, you've got nothing to worry about, right?"
Joe says, "Right."
Moe says, "Well if you get sent overseas you still got nothing to worry about. You'll either get sent to the front lines or not, right?" (During WWII the rear areas behind the front lines were relatively safe.)
Joe says, "Right."
Moe says, "Well if you don't get sent to the front you got nothing to worry about, right?"
Joe says, "Right."
Moe says, "Well if you do get sent to the front, you either get shot at or don't get shot at, right?"
Joe says, "Right."
Moe says, "Well if you don't get shot at you got nothing to worry about, right?"
Joe says, "Right."

Moe says, "Well if you do get shot at you still got nothing to worry about, you either get hit or you don't get hit, right?"

Joe says, "Right."

Moe says, "Well if you do get hit you still got nothing to worry about; you either get sent to the rear and recover and get to go home, or you don't recover and you die, right?"

Joe says, "Right."

Moe says, "Well if you recover and get to go home you've got nothing to worry about right?"

Joe says, "Right."

Moe says, "Well if you don't recover and die you've still got nothing to worry about, you either go to heaven or hell, right?"

Joe says, "Right."

Moe says, "Well if you go to heaven you've got nothing to worry about, right?"

Joe says, "Right."

Moe says, "Well if you go to hell you've still got nothing to worry about cause there is nothing you can do about it, right?"

Joe says, "Right," and decided to quit worrying.

Chapter 16:
Tools for Worry Management

1. Worry time: set a specific time to worry each day; and you must worry for at least 30 minutes.
2. Have a worry journal: write down everything you worry about in the journal.
3. If at any other time of day you start to obsess/worry about something, pull a rubber band back on your wrist and snap it and say, "Stop, it's not my worry time." Then take a deep breath, exhale slowly, tell yourself to relax, and then get back on task.

Exercise

Exercise is critically important. Kids do it naturally but most of us get out of the habit as we grow into adulthood and have jobs and families. There just doesn't seem to be enough time in the busy day. The chronic-pain patient has too much time. They are in too much pain to work, but also too much pain to do most sports. So what can you do? First get rid of the axiom of "no pain no gain." That may be fine for athletes but is wrong-headed for people who are already suffering severe pain. You don't want to do anything that will make your pain worse. Unfortunately, I've heard that some physical therapists say that their patients need to work through the pain. What morons. Also get rid of the guilt-ridden work ethic and thoughts that you should be doing something useful. You are doing something useful, you're taking care of yourself; you're gradually reconditioning yourself to your life with pain.

There are many options for types of exercise you can do just sitting in a chair or even when lying in bed. You have to find what works for you. I think that the most important thing to remember is to start slowly and work up very gradually. I ride a stationary bike, which I can program to automatically change the resistance while I ride. I usually read books while I ride and/or watch some television. Before I was hurt I usually rode at least 60 minutes almost every day and sometimes I'd ride 90 to 120 minutes. Since my injury, I was limited by my pain and lack of conditioning but still often rode for 45 to 60 minutes. This was before I finally figured out that it was that very act of bending over the handlebars of the bike that originally caused my injury by bending over my computer. Exercising gets your heart rate up and blood circulating; carrying oxygen to the cells and helping get rid of the build-up of toxic hormones that come from chronic pain/ stress. Remember I told you I switched to a stair stepper after years of exacerbating my back injury by bending over while riding.

If you're going to walk, get some good stable shoes—though I've known people who walk miles in just slippers. They don't have to be the expensive type. Most of the MDs I have seen stressed the need for me to walk rather than to ride my bike, as sitting on the bike compressed my spine more than walking. So, I started walking but developed some severe metatarsal pain in both feet. My orthopod suggested I try getting some MBT (*Masai* barefoot trainer) shoes. I did and they are wonderful, they have a curved bottom that takes a lot of the pressure off of the metatarsal joints. They are not inexpensive though—over $150—so this is not for everyone.

It may help you to have a walking buddy and/or group and find a place where it is safe to walk. As a motivator, keep a log of the times and distances you've walked so you can see the progress you make over time. You'll find a thousand excuses not to do it but you'll feel better if you do. It gives you a feeling of accomplishment and it is a critical part of weight management. Other types of exercises you can do include swimming, and/or walking in a pool, yoga, or any of the numerous types of oriental slow-movement exercises such as Tai Chi or Qui Chong. They may look simple but if you do them you'll find that they can quickly get your heart rate up, and you can do some of them sitting down.

DO SOMETHING. But start out with very small amounts and gradually expand the time as your body adjusts to the exercise.

Stretching is important both before and after exercising and can even be exercising in its own right.

Chapter 17:
Other Tools

Eating

Eating is one of the great pleasures of life; the tastes, aromas, and presentation. We almost all have some type of favorite comfort foods. Foods we eat when we're feeling sad or blue or down, and if you're in severe, chronic pain you certainly feel all of those. My favorites are macaroni and cheese, peanut butter and mayo sandwiches, a rich, creamy lemon chicken rice soup, and of course, the good old standbys of candy, candy bars, hard candies, cookies, blueberry muffins, and fresh baked bread. The obvious problem with comfort foods is that after you eat too much of them—and most of us do—you start to gain weight, especially with the decreased activity caused by your pain. It's another vicious cycle, you feel bad so you eat and the more you eat the worse you feel—guilt—so the more you eat.

Some five years prior to the start of my own chronic pain, I had decided that enough is enough when I reached 226 pounds and I'm only 5 feet 7 inches tall. As a youth and young man I had always been slender with a swimmer's body. My weight-management program, as I got past middle age, was to "buy bigger pants." In fact, that is going to be the title of my next book, *Buy Bigger Pants: Dr. Pollard's Miracle Weight-loss Program*. As I got heavier and wider around the waist, I'd just buy a bigger size of pants and bigger shirts. Fortunately, in Hawaii most men wear Aloha shirts, which are very loose fitting and can easily hide a lot of weight.

When I made the decision to stop, I didn't do anything radical, I just ate smaller portions and did more exercise, small things like walking three, then four, then five, then six flights of stairs two to three times a day and increased my bike riding. I did these increases gradually over time and the weight gradually came off. In about 18 months I had gone down to 170 and maintained my weight in that area—plus or minus a few pounds—for several years until my back became so severely painful. Then I went back to over 206 pounds before I again said pain or no pain, I'm happier with less weight and I have gradually been able to maintain near 170. Yet eating is one of those simple pleasures from which I encourage you to take more pleasure. Don't just eat the food for fuel or comfort, stop and savor each mouthful, taste the coffee, or tea, or lemon water. You're not in any rush to get anywhere. What do you have to do, finish eating quickly so that you can spend more time feeling your pain? Take the time to enjoy the pleasures of eating and drinking. Eat less and enjoy it more. Make that a mantra.

Music

Research has shown that listening to 20 minutes of music is as effective as taking medium—to high-strength pain medication to relieve pain. If I recall correctly it didn't matter what kind of music but I think it would have to be something you liked. My choice would be classical and/or country, "I'm tired of hanging my heart on your barbed-wire fence . . ." In my waiting room I have soft incandescent low lighting and music from either "A Walk in the Forest" or from "Pitta." Many patients tell me that they come to their appointments early just so that they can sit quietly and listen to the music and relax. I'm a one-person operation so there is usually only one person at a time sitting in my waiting room.

One of my patients is bothered by severe tinnitus—a ringing in the ears—and finds that listening to music on headphones masks the ringing and makes his life more bearable. I got him in touch with the National Tinnitus Society for other suggestions.

We don't know why music helps relieve pain. My hypothesis is that while the brain is processing the music, it is distracted from the pain signals. Of course there are times when listening to music just doesn't cut it and I need my pain medication and I need it NOW. "Listen to music, you gotta be kidding Doc. What you smoking?"

Again it's just another tool that some people find helpful.

Laughter/Humor

As the *Reader's Digest* says, "Laughter is the best medicine." Again there is research to support that claim. A good belly laugh that almost causes you to cry, releases endorphins in the blood stream which help lessen the pain. So look for humor and laugh at yourself and at life. What's the alternative? To cry? Read the cartoons and ask people to tell you jokes. Look up humor in your library and/or on the Internet and subscribe to a humor newsletter. Watch the comedy channel on TV; rent funny videos. I've seen Abbott and Costello's, "Who's on First?" skit dozens of times and still get chuckles each time I watch it.

You have to be old enough to remember Abbott and Costello, and too old to REALLY understand computers, to fully appreciate the one below. For those of us who sometimes get flustered by our computers, please read on . . . If Bud Abbott and Lou Costello were alive today, their famous sketch, "Who's on First?" might have turned out something like this:

COSTELLO CALLS TO BUY A COMPUTER FROM ABBOTT

ABBOTT: Super Duper computer store. Can I help you?

COSTELLO: Thanks. I'm setting up an office in my den and I'm thinking about buying a computer.

ABBOTT: Mac?

COSTELLO: No, the name's Lou.

ABBOTT: Your computer?

COSTELLO: I don't own a computer. I want to buy one.

ABBOTT: Mac?

COSTELLO: I told you, my name's Lou.

ABBOTT: What about Windows?

COSTELLO: Why? Will it get stuffy in here?

ABBOTT: Do you want a computer with Windows?

COSTELLO: I don't know. What will I see when I look at the windows?

ABBOTT: Wallpaper.

COSTELLO: Never mind the windows. I need a computer and software.

ABBOTT: Software for Windows?

COSTELLO: No. On the computer! I need something I can use to write proposals and track expenses and run my business. What do you have?

ABBOTT: Office.

COSTELLO: Yeah, for my office. Can you recommend anything?

ABBOTT: I just did.

COSTELLO: You just did what?

ABBOTT: Recommend something.

COSTELLO: You recommended something?

ABBOTT: Yes.

COSTELLO: For my office?

ABBOTT: Yes.

COSTELLO: OK, what did you recommend for my office?

ABBOTT: Office.

COSTELLO: Yes, for my office!

ABBOTT: I recommend Office with Windows.

COSTELLO: I already have an office with windows! OK, let's just say I'm sitting at my computer and I want to type a proposal. What do I need?

ABBOTT: Word.

COSTELLO: What word?

ABBOTT: Word in Office.

COSTELLO: The only word in office is office.

ABBOTT: The Word in Office for Windows.

COSTELLO: Which word in office for windows?

ABBOTT: The Word you get when you click on the blue "W."

COSTELLO: I'm going to click your blue "w" if you don't start with some straight answers. What about financial bookkeeping? You have anything I can track my money with?

ABBOTT: Money.

COSTELLO: That's right. What do you have?

ABBOTT: Money.

COSTELLO: I need money to track my money?

ABBOTT: It comes bundled with your computer.

COSTELLO: What's bundled with my computer?

ABBOTT: Money . . .

COSTELLO: Money comes with my computer?

ABBOTT: Yes. No extra charge.

COSTELLO: I get a bundle of money with my computer? How much?

ABBOTT: One copy.

COSTELLO: Isn't it illegal to copy money?

ABBOTT: Microsoft gave us a license to copy Money.

COSTELLO: They can give you a license to copy money?

ABBOTT: Why not? THEY OWN IT!

(A few days later)

ABBOTT: Super Duper computer store. Can I help you?

COSTELLO: How do I turn my computer off?

ABBOTT: Click on "START."

The humor I like the best is the real-life stuff, funny directions, like "Don't put hand under lawn mower while running." Duh, you think. Or actual computer tech reports:

Subject: Tech support

Tech support: What kind of computer do you have?

Female customer: A white one . . .

===============

Customer: Hi, this is Celine. I can't get my diskette out.

Tech support: Have you tried pushing the button?

Customer: Yes, sure, it's really stuck.

Tech support: That doesn't sound good; I'll make a note.

Customer: No . . . wait a minute . . . I hadn't inserted it yet . . . it's still on my desk . . . sorry . . .

===============

Tech support: Click on the "My Computer" icon on the left of the screen.

Customer: Your left or my left?

===============

Tech support: Good day. How may I help you?

Male customer: Hello . . . I can't print.

Tech support: Would you click on "Start" for me and . . .

Customer: Listen pal; don't start getting technical on me! I'm not Bill Gates, dammit!

===============

Customer: Hi, good afternoon, this is Martha, I can't print. Every time I try, it says "Can't find printer." I've even lifted the printer and placed it in front of the monitor, but the computer still says he can't find it . . .

================

Customer: I have problems printing in red . . .
Tech support: Do you have a color printer?
Customer: Aaaah . . . . thank you.

================

Tech support: What's on your monitor now, ma'am?
Customer: A teddy bear my boyfriend bought for me at the 7-11.

================

Customer: My keyboard is not working anymore.
Tech support: Are you sure it's plugged into the computer?
Customer: No. I can't get behind the computer.
Tech support: Pick up your keyboard and walk 10 paces back.
Customer: OK.
Tech support: Did the keyboard come with you?
Customer: Yes.
Tech support: That means the keyboard is not plugged in. Is there another keyboard?
Customer: Yes, there's another one here. Ah . . . that one does work . . .

===============

Tech support: Your password is the small letter "a" as in "apple", a capital letter "V" as in "Victor", the number 7.

Customer: Is that 7 in capital letters?

===============

Customer: I can't get on the Internet.

Tech support: Are you sure you used the right password?

Customer: Yes, I'm sure. I saw my colleague do it.

Tech support: Can you tell me what the password was?

Customer: Five stars.

===============

Tech support: What anti-virus program do you use?

Customer: Netscape.

Tech support: That's not an anti-virus program.

Customer: Oh, sorry . . . Internet Explorer.

===============

Customer: I have a huge problem. A friend has placed a screen saver on my computer, but every time I move the mouse, it disappears.

===============

Tech support: How may I help you?

Customer: I'm writing my first e-mail.

Tech support: OK, and what seems to be the problem?

Customer: Well, I have the letter "a" in the address, but how do I get the circle around it?

================

A woman customer called the Canon help desk with a problem with her printer.

Tech support: Are you running it under windows?

Customer: No, my desk is next to the door, but that is a good point. The man sitting in the cubicle next to me is under a window, and his printer is working fine.

================

And last but not least . . .

Tech support: Okay Bob, let's press the control and escape keys at the same time. That brings up a task list in the middle of the screen. Now type the letter "P" to bring up the "Program Manager."

Customer: I don't have a P.

Tech support: On your keyboard, Bob.

Customer: What do you mean?

Tech support: "P" . . . on your keyboard, Bob.

Customer: I'M NOT GOING TO DO THAT!

Whew. I got a good laugh out of re-reading those.

Or how about testimony from actual trials? These are from a book titled, *Disorder in the American Courts*, and are things people actually said in court, word for word, taken down and now published by court reporters who had the torment of staying calm while these exchanges were actually taking place.

ATTORNEY: Are you sexually active?
WITNESS: No, I just lie there.

ATTORNEY: What was the first thing your husband said to you that morning?
WITNESS: He said, "Where am I, Cathy?"
ATTORNEY: And why did that upset you?
WITNESS: My name is Susan.

ATTORNEY: Now doctor, isn't it true that when a person dies in his sleep, he doesn't know about it until the next morning?
WITNESS: Did you actually pass the bar exam?

ATTORNEY: Do you recall the time that you examined the body?
WITNESS: The autopsy started around 8:30 p.m.
ATTORNEY: And Mr. Denton was dead at the time?

WITNESS: No, he was sitting on the table wondering why I was doing an autopsy on him!

AND THE WINNER GOES TO . . .

ATTORNEY: Doctor, before you performed the autopsy, did you check for a pulse?

WITNESS: No.

ATTORNEY: Did you check for blood pressure?

WITNESS: No.

ATTORNEY: Did you check for breathing?

WITNESS: No.

ATTORNEY: So, then it is possible that the patient was alive when you began the autopsy?

WITNESS: No.

ATTORNEY: How can you be so sure, Doctor?

WITNESS: Because his brain was sitting on my desk in a jar.

ATTORNEY: But could the patient have still been alive, nevertheless?

WITNESS: Yes, it is possible that he could have been alive and practicing law.

I hope you get the point. Make a humor file and refer to it often. If you like these, buy the book, as I've just given you a few examples.

Norman Cousins became famous for his book, *Anatomy of an Illness*. He told the story of his life and how he had been diagnosed with an incurable, very painful connective-tissue disease and was given six months to live. He got off all of his medications and devoted hours and hours to watching old funny movies—he also took mega doses of vitamin C—and credits his life being saved by his laughter. It's a great book.

TV/DVDs/Reading

Thank God and/or the inventors for making TV, cable, and DVDs. Chronic-pain patients need all the distractions they can get. My evenings have been reduced to watching funny old DVDs from Netflix. I'm too tired and in too much pain to do much of anything else. But that's putting it in a negative frame. What I need to say is that my pain has given me the opportunity to watch so many DVDs and TV shows that I wouldn't have otherwise had the time to watch. I love "Northern Exposure", "The Gods Must Be Crazy", "Columbo", "Faulty Towers", "Waiting for God", and many others. It doesn't take my pain away but it does distract me for a few hours.

The same can be said for reading, and books from the library are free, well except for gas there and back, and they have books in big print for my old eyes or even audio books and DVDs to rent for a dollar a week. I can get into a good murder mystery or detective story and be gone for hours. Sometimes this is not so good, I may stay up late just to finish a book and then my sleep cycle is all messed up the next day and I get mad at myself—guilt again—for not being more productive and wasting time.

See how that keeps coming up again and again, guilt, which creates tension, which makes my pain worse. Stop it!

Like all things, watching TV, DVDs, and/or reading needs to be balanced with the rest of your life and in some moderation, but there is no reason not to enjoy them as a tool for coping with your pain. You can tell your spouse, "Dr. Pollard said so."

One warning about TV, if you're a news junky you may be stressing yourself out and making your pain worse. There is so much violence, hatred, and tragedy in the world. You, I, can get all worked up and stressed out about things we can't change. And what does that do for your pain? So it might be a good idea to limit your news watching or schedule your worry time right after the news. The same can be said about books. I only read books that I'm pretty sure have a happy ending—sometimes I actually read the end first to make sure it's going to be okay—and won't read any books that involve children being harmed or hurt in any way.

If you don't know where your local library is, find out, get a library card, and use it. Your library is your friend; you can be alone and yet around people. If you don't have access to a computer and the Internet, the library does, and it's usually free. They are required to be accessible to the disabled. They have people who will help you and show you how to get online and do research. Take a pillow with you as the chair may be a little hard. They are usually very tolerant of pain patients needing to stand and pace without booting them off the computer. Anything you want, you can find on the Internet if you know how to look. Don't be afraid to try. Don't forget to take your emergency pain pills with you.

Internet

What a wonderful world we live in. If you're fortunate enough to have a computer and access to the Internet you have a whole new world to explore. You can look up anything. It's like a huge library that never closes and is always open and there are no restricted sections. Again you need to do it in moderation and balance it with the rest of your life—what life dummy? I'm in constant pain. Okay so forget it . . . Not. Through the Internet you can join emotional support groups, play role-playing games, and share email with people all over the world. And you can research your particular type of pain or disease.

I use it mostly for emailing and for shopping online. It's just easier to do than driving to a store. And it's fun.

There is a certain sense of peace and control to be able to type in a chat room or type an email at any time of the day or night. It makes new types of pen pals, instantly communicating or even chatting real-time with video. You also have to learn what email tricks to watch out for so that you aren't bilked out of thousands of dollars. There is so much of the world to explore, whatever your interests are; you can find it on the Internet. You can join common interest groups. And before you know it, hours and hours have gone by and you haven't been as aware of your pain.

You can write books and if you can't type there are even programs that convert your spoken words into typed text. You can send your recorded thoughts on Blogs and even make your own video and post it on Youtube. Wikipedia, the free Internet encyclopedia, defines blog: (a contraction of the term "weblog") a type of website, usually maintained by an individual with regular entries of commentary, descriptions of events, or other material such as graphics or video. Entries are commonly displayed in reverse chronological order. "Blog" can also be used as a verb, meaning to maintain or add content to a blog.

Many blogs provide commentary or news on a particular subject; others function as more personal online diaries. A typical blog combines text, images, and links to other blogs, web pages, and other media related to its topic. The ability for readers to leave comments in an interactive format is an important part of many blogs. Most blogs are primarily textual, although some focus on art (artlog), photographs (photoblog), sketches (sketchblog), videos (vlog), music (MP3 blog), and audio (podcasting). Micro-blogging is another type of blogging, featuring very short posts. As of December 2007, the blog search engine Technorati was tracking more than 112 million blogs. The Internet world awaits you at any time you choose. But be careful as there are some things that seem very innocent and safe which are really traps trolling for the unwary user. I haven't even mentioned Twittering or Face Book which is mostly how the younger generation communicates with each other. Don't think you're too old to learn.

Sex

News flash; sex is wonderful. Not just the orgasm but the cuddling and closeness that comes with it. When you have it you don't know how much you'll miss it when it's gone. Orgasms are a wonderful, wonderful whole-being feeling of deep pleasure. They release hormones that are natural painkillers. GREAT if you can have them.

Unfortunately, chronic, severe pain often leaves one unable to have sex. It just hurts too much. And even if it doesn't hurt too much, the side effects of many of the medications, *Neuronton*, *Lyrica*, anti-depressants, and pain medications—to name a few—leave one just uninterested in sex. For a man, even if you manage to have some interest and get an erection, you can't ejaculate. And that is frustrating. Again, speaking for men, many men feel guilty for not being able to pleasure their mates and feel a loss of their very manhood, which leads to more depression and stress and worse pain. Another vicious cycle. The greater the pleasure you had from sex before the chronic pain, the more you miss it when it's gone. It's another one of those things that you can't do that you used to be able to do. Damn! F*** it, no can't do that. #%@**.

Women also feel shame and guilt that they can't please their mate, but since I'm not a woman I can't speak in any depth about how it is or isn't for them. Some feel guilty and some use it as an acceptable excuse to not have to have sex. Both males and females fear the potential loss of their mate and they need to be able to have frank and honest talks about these fears. The same as men, women fear the loss of their womanhood.

If you live alone this problem of sex is less important than if you live with someone with whom you were used to being sexually intimate. It takes a while, but over time you can learn that it just isn't the be all and end all of the totally highest priority in life. You can live happily without it . . . not. The solutions are many and varied, but key to it is being able to communicate with your mate without guilt, or shame, or blame about your sexual needs or lack of them, and their needs and how you can help each other.

The sex drive is somewhat like the need for water, food, and air; you have to have them to survive. But you can live without sex. Some men and women choose to live a life of celibacy. Freud, however, would have said that they are, in reality, repressing or sublimating their sex drives, and these drives will come out in some other way. I think Freud is both right and wrong. He was right that it is a strong biological urge, but wrong in that not everyone has it, or the same amount of it. I know that most, but not all, the men I see in treatment miss it. I surprised myself when I began to not miss it, but cuddling and physical closeness is very nice even without sex. Many women, on the other hand, say they can live happily without it.

"The self is only that which is in the process of becoming" (Kierkegaard).

Guilt-Free Depression

Of course you're depressed because of the severe, constant pain and the loss of being able to do most of the things you used to do. Who wouldn't be depressed? If you tell me you're never depressed, you're really good at lying to yourself or you're not really in that much pain, or you've reached that stage of chronic pain called acceptance—but that comes and goes.

All of my chronic-pain patients are more or less depressed at least some of the time—not necessarily suicidal—but they don't want to live with the pain and loss of function and say that they would be happy if they just didn't wake up one morning. Fortunately for me and their families, none of them have killed themselves. And of course the depression makes you feel guilty, and then tense, and then the pain is worse, and you're more depressed.

Cheer up. Life is good. Yeah easy for you to say. Not so easy to do.

One of the ways I use to help people cope with this depression is to write them a prescription to be depressed for 24 hours, guilt free. In the state of Hawaii, psychologists are not licensed to write prescriptions for medications. Nonetheless, I have my prescription pad and I write them a behavioral prescription to be depressed for 24 hours guilt free, to be refilled PRN—that's medical talk for as needed—but not more than one day a week. Sometimes I have to give them more than one day a week. I tell them to stay in bed, cry, pull the covers over their head, and feel sorry for themselves, and if anyone asks they can show them their Doctor's prescription. By telling them that it is okay and giving them a prescription in writing from a doctor, they can be depressed—which they are going to be anyway—but without the guilt, and without the guilt they don't feel as depressed and tense, and the pain is less. Then the next day they get up and get back on track with their life; wherever that is.

You can laugh, but it works. Something about an authority—"The Doctor"—giving you written permission frees the person from the guilt and responsibility.

Anger/Emotional Management

"Am I angry? Duh, you think? You f***ing bet I am. I want to hurt those bastards and make them feel the way I feel. They don't care about me. It's just the money to them. F*** them. I'll show them what hurt is. F***ing #@**-heads. They're not the one who can't work or pay their bills. What? You're f***ing stupid, asking me if I'm angry. *#*^&**." On and on goes the litany of angry words and thoughts. Anger is one of the recurring stages of pain. It is natural and normal. Who wouldn't be angry in chronic, severe pain? It is also—over time—one of the most self-destructive emotions.

While it is normal to feel angry and to vent it appropriately, it becomes pathological and destructive if you dwell in the house of anger. It starts the vicious cycle over again; anger creates tension, which makes the pain worse, which leads to more anger. And round and round it goes.

So if it is normal how do you deal with it? What causes the anger? It's the pain, right? Wrong, partly. The pain causes pain but it's what you tell yourself about the pain and the loss of function that causes the anger. It's your thoughts that cause the anger to continue. The anger may start with the pain, but if you continue to dwell on the negative thoughts about the pain and all of your losses, then you are the one who is making yourself angry.

Some of my patients say, "Oh, I get it Doc. I'm letting it make me angry." And I say, "May I make a correction in your thinking?" They say, "Yes."

"When you say you let it or allowed it to make you angry, you're still putting the blame or responsibility for your anger out there on 'it' whatever 'it' is. You are not taking responsibility by passively implying that you let it make you angry. No. You made yourself angry. How? By telling yourself negative things about the pain and loss. It's a lot different to say, 'I'm making myself angry,' rather than, 'I'm letting it make me angry.'"

What are the negative thoughts? That's what you have to identify. Complete the sentence, "I'm angry because . . ." Anything that comes after the "because" is self-talk or thoughts about the pain and loss. It is those thoughts which you have to identify and change if you are really going to learn—emphasis on the word learn—to manage your anger and other emotions more effectively. Who does your anger hurt the most? You, and those around you.

I give my patients a handout on "Anger and Emotional Management." This is certainly not original from me. In various forms it has been a staple of cognitive behavioral therapy for 60 or more years.

This section may sound academic and boring but it is critically necessary if you are really going to learn how to control the strong emotions that come as part of the deal when you were selected to have chronic, severe pain. This is very hard work and usually takes my patients weeks or months—regardless of how smart or educated they may be—to come to a real understanding of the process so that they can use it as an effective tool.

To manage strong emotions of anger and/or hurt, which always accompany chronic, severe pain, you may first need to take a cool down away from the person or situation or pain. The cool down starts with a deep breath, slowly exhaling, while telling yourself to relax. Then using one of the coping tools. This cool down needs to last long enough for you to do a "think down" to understand how your thinking has led to your emotion, and how changing your thinking about the situation and pain, and/or person will change your emotions, actions, and results.

When you're in chronic, severe pain you feel like swearing. This is when you may need to use this SWEWEAR acronym—each letter stands for part of the process of managing your emotions. In a journal make **SWEWEAR** entries as indicated below. You can just use the letter in parentheses ( ) for each heading. This process is to help you understand when you feel like "swearing" due to your pain or for any reason, how your self-talk about a situation or pain leads to your feelings and actions, and the results of your actions. You may need to read through this two or three times to understand how this will help you learn to control your emotions. It took me a couple of years to learn and that was long before I developed my own severe, chronic pain.

(S) SITUATION: What happened, what was going on? This should be only as long as necessary to describe what happened. It should be a "snapshot" of the event and should be only observable **facts.** If you use the word "because" to describe the situation, anything after the word "because" is self-talk and belongs under W1.

Example:
(1) My spouse was supposed to meet me for dinner at a local restaurant at 6 PM but she never showed up.

(W1) WHAT YOU TELL YOURSELF first: What you are telling yourself about the situation—not facts, but your **opinions**? What you are thinking? What meaning do you put on the event?

Example:
(1) Who the fuck does he/she think he/she is? I'm humiliated and embarrassed. He/she always does this. He/she doesn't care about me. It's not fair. I can't stand it when this happens. He/she knows it

makes my pain worse to have to wait around.

(E1) EMOTION 1: What you **feel.** Just two to three words.

Example:

(1) Anger, pissed off, hurt, in pain.

(W2) WHAT YOU TELL YOURSELF 2 (SELF-TALK 2): Counter or change everything (line by line) you told yourself in W1.

Example:

(1) Who he/she thinks they are is not the issue. Whether or not I'm humiliated and/or embarrassed is not the issue. Whether it is the third or fifth time is not the issue. Whether or not he/she cares about me is not the issue. Whether or not it is fair or not is not the issue. Whether she knows it makes my pain worse or not is not the issue. The issue is that I'm not going to **continue** to make myself upset or angry by thinking these negative thoughts. I'm going to breathe and cool down and write a SWEWEAR.

(E2) EMOTION 2: What you feel now after countering your negative self-talk (W1).

Example:
(1) calm.
ACTION(A): What you **did**.

Example:
(1) I used an "I" message to talk to him/her about my feelings and thoughts about showing up when we agreed to and I used active listening to hear her side. I wrote a SWEWEAR.

(RRR) RESULT/REACTION/RESPONSE: What happened as a result or as a response to your action? What was the result for you?

Example:
(1) I felt good by using "I" messages to tell him/her how I felt and using active listening we came to an agreement about meeting when we say we will. I didn't stay angry and my pain decreased.

This process of recognizing and changing your self-talk is very difficult and is like learning a new language. The more you practice it the easier it gets and the better you get at managing your emotions. Your emotions come from your thinking about the pain. ONLY when you are emotionally calm, can you engage in problem-solving communication with your spouse or family or friends.

I also give the following handout to most of my patients who are having problems with getting mad at other people, and certainly if you are in severe pain you will be getting mad.

"The Sun Rises in the East": A Logical Thinking, Anger-Management Tool

1. Do you get angry because the sun rises in the East rather than the West? Of course not—there is no reason to get angry at the sun rising in the East; that is just the way it is. There is no need or usefulness at getting angry at things that are a certain way. It makes no sense to get angry at this.
2. It is a fact of life that all human beings do things we shouldn't do and don't do all the things we should do. That is the way we are; it is a fact of life, just like the sun rising in the East.
3. Therefore it makes no sense to get angry at people when they do or don't do things they should or shouldn't do. They are not making you mad or irritated; you are making yourself angry by illogically telling yourself that they shouldn't be the way they

are. Maybe they shouldn't, but that is the way they are, and you can't change them any more than you can change where the sun rises. Your irritation/anger only hurts you and those around you.

4. Take a really deep breath, exhale very slowly, and tell yourself to relax. Then counter your self-talk about what people should or shouldn't do and say to yourself, "The sun rises in the East." Accept life as it is.

5. When you have calmed down and let go of your irritation/anger then you may be able to do some rational thinking to find a solution to the problem of what someone is or isn't doing without your irritation/anger getting in the way.

"Freedom is within each of us. What happens outside is of little consequence." Source: Margaret Truman in *Murder at the FBI*.

Fake it till you make it

Attitude can be everything, and it sends ripples out all around us. If your attitude is negative it will have negative effects for you and others. If your attitude is positive it will have positive effects for you and others. You have a choice about what kind of attitude you will have each hour and each day. I didn't say it would be easy—especially when the pain is bad—but you still have a choice. Think of the power of thought: a golfer teas up his ball and says to his buddies, "I'll probably slice this one." He is actually setting his mind to have his body slice the shot and sure enough he does.

Even if you're frustrated and irritated, put on a happy face and act like you are happy and after a while you begin to actually feel happy. Or as Shakespeare put it: "Assume the virtue if you have it not."

Numerous books have been written about the power of positive thinking. You've got to get rid of "I can't do it," and think instead, "I'm going to learn how." Google "power of positive thinking" and get a book and read it.

Examples in medicine almost make it the rule rather than the exception. The doctor tells a boy that he'll never walk again and the boy is determined to show the doctor he is wrong and guess what? The boy learns to walk again. One woman I've worked with was so badly injured that the doctors told her she'd never be able to go back to work and would have to have someone to take care of her for the rest of her life. It took her more than four years, but she had a very determined attitude and she is now back to work. She sent a letter to the doctors chastising them for telling her she would never be able to do it. They should have given her some hope, however slim.

Do you remember the children's book about the *Little Train That Could*? The train repeats to itself over and over as it is trying to climb a steep hill, "I think I can, I think I can, I think I can." If you tell yourself you can't, then you can't, and there is no need to even try. Just give up. I know, sometimes I/you feel that way but we have to get out of it; the alternative is a *Dead Life* or a life that is *Dead*.

Another form of faking it is to take a trip. When you're gone away from home and the community, no one knows you, and universally my chronic-pain patients tell me how pleasant and therapeutic it is to get away from all the worries, even if just for a little while, and even if they are still in pain. During the time of the trip they could forget about all the legal and insurance company problems and live a better life even with the pain. Unfortunately—there's that word again—when they come back they can feel all that emotional stress and trauma weighing them down again. It's like when you're gone away it's easier to do the first part of the Serenity Prayer, "Grant me the serenity to accept the things I cannot change . . ."

The trip doesn't have to be long in terms of distance away from home or how long you're away, but for a little while you're completely away from all the stresses, phone calls, letters, and doctors' appointments.

Examples abound in the field of athletics of the power of the mind. In one study of basketball players shooting free throws, two groups were divided up, matched in their average percentage of free-throw accuracy. One group practiced doing actual free throws 30 minutes a day for a month. The other group didn't do any actual practice of shooting free throws but instead practiced in their minds imagining successfully shooting free throws. As you probably guessed by now, the mind practice group did the same as or better than the actual practice group.

There isn't any sport, from golf to platform diving, that doesn't have a huge component of mental practice and/or imaging that separates the great from all the rest. Tiger Woods is a prime example. Professional divers practice and review all of their body movements in their minds before they ever do the actual dive. I could give you many more examples but the purpose is not tell you about sports but rather to show you how important your mental outlook and attitude are in how you cope with your pain.

Sleeping

When you sleep well your body and mind have a chance to recharge and rebuild. Lack of sleep makes everything worse. It makes you tense, grouchy, and the pain is then worse. So how do you get a good night's sleep? It has been my experience that each person has to find their own unique way of shutting down the mind and relaxing the body so that they can sleep. Some people like a warm glass of milk just before bed and lights out. I like to read for an hour or two to take my mind off of the worries/activities of the day. However, if it is a good detective story I sometimes find myself staying up late because I want to find out what happens next. I have to remind myself to turn out the light and let myself go to sleep. I always look at the clock just before I turn out the lights and I tell myself that if I'm not asleep within 30 minutes, I'll get up and do some relaxation exercises and/or take some medicine. What you don't want to do is lie in bed awake for hours trying to get to sleep. If you can't sleep, get up and do something, and then, after an hour or so you can try again to sleep.

Some people are very afraid to sleep because of the nightmares of past events in their life that they relive over and over again in their dreams. They literally are terrified of going to sleep. For this you might try processing those events in psychotherapy and/or using a combination of medications for anxiety and sleep and consider natural herbs.

I currently take sleep medication on a nightly basis. I have taken *Restoril*, *Lunesta*, *Ambien CR*, *Valium*, *Amitriptyline*, and *Soma,* and sometimes a prophylactic hydrocodone pill. It is good to have different medications so that if your body becomes acclimated or tolerant of a certain medication, and it is no longer working, you can switch to a different medication.

Some people say not to exercise before bed and others say exercise before bed helps them sleep. The same is true about eating a big meal late at night just before going to bed. Some find a short walk before bed helps. You have to find what works for you.

Is your bed too hard or too soft? In the past hard beds or mattresses even with a bed-board under them were prescribed for back-pain sufferers. Recent research in a Danish study, reported in *USA Weekend*, found that people with chronic low-back pain, who slept on water beds or a body-conforming foam mattress, reported less pain and nearly an hour more sleep a night than those who slept on a hard futon mattress. There are many types of mattress and many commercials claiming that their particular product will give you a good night's sleep. Unfortunately, they cost thousands of dollars. I have been able to make my own multilayered memory foam type of mattress for under $200. Still, some nights, the pain overpowers any sleep medications and the next day is compromised. And that is part of having chronic, severe pain. I wish I had a magic solution to give you. Do some research on the Internet and try different things until you find something that works for you.

Paradoxical Intention

Don't worry. Cheer up. Don't be so depressed. *"That's easy for you to say Doc,"* the patients think. When all the straightforward approaches to getting people to manage their pain effectively don't seem to be working, I pull out what I call my "big gun", "paradoxical intention." It's one of the most powerful tools a therapist has.

Paradoxical intention is the opposite of what you want. So if I've tried to cheer someone up using many of the coping strategies I talk about in this book and they're not getting any better, I tell they something like, "Well, it looks like you haven't suffered enough yet. I think we need to set a goal for you to suffer and be depressed at least 12 hours a day and if that doesn't work we can go up to 18 hours a day and that ought to work."

At this point the patient usually looks at me with a questioning expression, like did they hear me correctly? I say, "Yeah, I just don't think you've suffered enough yet. Maybe we should start at 14 hours a day and remember no smiling or laughing. You're to feel bad, rotten, for the whole time." Usually by this time they are beginning to smile or laugh, and I say, "Hey. No laughing. You've got to take this more seriously."

It might not seem funny reading it on paper but it works. It has to be done with some skill and finesse and only after extensive listening and trying other things. Sometimes it takes me a while before I get the person to smile; I have to really lay it on thick like, "You know you're the worst person I've ever run into in all my years of practice. I may have to write a paper about your depression and suffering. I bet we could get you in the *Guinness Book of World Records*." On occasion I have wondered if I'm going to get them to catch on.

Then I go on and tell them what I'm doing. Most people call it trying to use reverse psychology on them but it works, even if they know what you're doing. I usually share some examples for them to relate to. It's like when a parent says to a child throwing a temper tantrum, "Can't you cry any louder than that?" But it has to be done in a matter of fact way and with some gentle humor. I will even give them a written prescription to be depressed and/or suffer at least 10 hours a day and to refill as needed.

Either way I've got them, got them to face what they are doing to themselves. If they follow my prescription then they are proving that they have a choice; if they don't follow directions then they have chosen to stop focusing on their suffering. When they are on the way out of my office I'll say something like, "Now remember no laughing or smiling. I'm going to want to know how much suffering you've done next time I see you."

The paradox is that by trying to suffer and/or feel depressed and worried even more than you are, the opposite happens; you suffer less, are less depressed, and less worried. My daughter even uses it on me.

We live in a great country where we are more or less guaranteed to have the right to life, liberty, and the pursuit of happiness. My own belief is that happiness is a byproduct of doing things that you like to do and/or that you need to do. Unfortunately, there are those few individuals who do want to suffer and won't give it up. But I usually don't see them because they're not really interested in coming to therapy—it might help.

Pain happens, but suffering is optional, or the amount of suffering you do is optional.

Hobbies/Games/Pets

Hobbies are a wonderful way to distract your mind from the pain and trials of living. Unfortunately, the injuries and pain may keep a person from enjoying the very hobbies that they used to love so much. Now you have to learn a new hobby or how to just watch others do the things you used to do and take vicarious pleasure from watching them. I have one patient who used to love to work on old cars and now he can't. But he has learned how to love teaching his son how to do it.

Playing physical games with children or grandchildren is often severely limited. You can't bounce them on your knee or play horsy or roll around on the floor with them. But you can play board games with them from almost any age and read books to them. You've got to be firm in setting limits on what you can do with them and when it's time to quit you need to quit.

If you've never had a hobby you might find it helpful to try to find one. Look for something that interests you, from photography to fly making. Join a group of people who have a similar interest. I know you don't want to go out but you need to, at least some of the time, and for at least a little while. Being around other people who are interested in something will motivate and stimulate you. Not you? Okay, back to suffering for you.

Pet therapy is actually a sub-type of psychotherapy, as is play therapy, and it's not just for children. Pets have been shown in numerous research studies to be very beneficial in improving mood and decreasing anxiety and the need for medication for pain and depression. Whether it is a dog or cat or some other animal, humans seem to derive a great deal of pleasure from having an animal to take care of who loves them unconditionally no matter how bad the day has been. Your dog will lick your face and your cat will crawl between your legs and nest in your lap. Other pets like fish or birds or hamsters are okay, but to me they don't seem to have the same amount and kind of interactions that dogs and cats do.

Some people don't want the burden of caring for a pet and that is all right. Each person has to find what helps them through the day. I would suggest that if you're thinking about getting a pet for a family member who is in pain that you need to talk to them first. They may really not want one.

Having pets in apartments or rental houses used to be a problem, but not now. I'm not an attorney but with the Americans with Disabilities Act, I think Federal law requires apartments, condominiums, and rental houses to not discriminate against pet owners if a doctor certifies that the pet is required as part of their medical treatment and therapy, in the same way that a blind person can have a seeing-eye dog go everywhere with them.

Many, if not most, of my chronic-pain patients have and love their dogs, or cats, or goats, or chickens.

Just another tool you might use.

Drinking

By all means drink plenty of water to keep hydrated. But what about drinking alcohol? All the prescriptions say not to drink any alcohol while taking this medication. Yet there is a lot of good research that says drinking one to two glasses of wine or one or two shots of liquor is good for your overall health. If you can drink one or two drinks and stop this may be something you may want to try. If you can't or don't stop at two then you probably shouldn't do this. It is your decision, as always, to make. Many of my chronic-pain patients do drink one or two drinks a day and find that it helps them. Again the choice is yours. I would suggest that you discuss it with your primary treating MD.

Chapter 18:
Purpose in Life

Without a purpose in life, goals and dreams, and things you want to do, life becomes meaningless and you really have no reason to live, to get up in the morning, and get going. Anecdotally you hear about it all the time. An elderly person or a sick person has a goal of living to see their daughter get married or their son graduate from college and once that goal is achieved they die. With no purpose you wallow in the quagmire of the pain process.

It's imperative for chronic, severe-pain patients to have some motivating purpose to keep them going, a reason to keep struggling to cope with the pain. It doesn't really matter what that purpose is as long as they have it. Unfortunately, most chronic-pain patients had a purpose and goals and dreams that have to be abandoned or drastically changed or completely redone because of the pain and subsequent loss of function.

One patient I treated had a goal of building his own solar-panel installation company, but now he can't get up on ladders, much less on roofs. He has, however, found a new interest in aquaculture and his eyes light up when he begins to talk about the possibilities. Another was a security guard, who was injured to the extent that psychologically he couldn't return to that line of work, but now he is very enthused about building a commercial organic-tomato farm.

I could go on and on. My point is that the pain patients who make progress at managing their pain are the ones who develop a new purpose in their lives. One took over the raising of her grandchildren. She can't do the heavy work but she still knows how to parent. When you have a purpose, you begin to make plans and think about how to make the purpose come to fruition. And then you're not in as much pain.

Initially, for the new patient with pain that will become chronic, the purpose is to cope with the pain on a day-to-day basis and this may last a long time. Eventually they need to get a purpose that is broader or larger than just their pain. I don't know specifically what your purpose will be, but you must find one. If you do you'll be a giant step ahead of millions of people who don't have any purpose. The injury and pain **gives you the opportunity** to travel in new directions and find a new purpose and meaning in your life. "F*** that. I want my old life back." Well back to suffering for you.

My situation is unique, as is everyone's. My purpose is the same as a chronic-pain patient as it was before, to help others through therapy, writing, and my paintings. The pain and the process of coping with it have made me a far better therapist, and not just for pain patients, but for all patients. All human problems are a type of pain and most of them are chronic whether an addiction, anxiety, depression, obsession, marital discord, or any of the other conditions for which people seek therapy. I'd like to see couples spend as much time planning their lives together as they do on planning the wedding. I hope to make this book available to pain patients at minimal or no cost. If someone likes one of my paintings and it really moves them, I'd like to give it to them, but reality has shown me I at least need to get some costs back. And unfortunately, our culture tends to devalue something if it is free, inferring that it must not be worth anything if it's free. The pain patient has to learn that the free things in life are some of the most important, like breathing clean air, drinking pure water, feeling the sun, wind, seeing the clouds, sky, trees, mountains, seas, flowers, and appreciating our loved ones, and even the stranger you meet standing in line.

I get up wishing I had more time to do more things. This has only been since I've been getting better, as before it was just to get through the night and then one hour at a time and one more day—to paint and write and see patients. I still have to do my back exercises, go to my various therapies and doctors' appointments, get my prescriptions filled, and do all of the activities of daily living we all have to do. My purpose is to enjoy all of these things in the moment they are happening, even as I type this.

One mother whose child had been killed by a drunk driver made it her purpose in life to start MADD, Mothers Against Drunk Driving. Become your own champion, focusing on the things that you can do. Let those things you can't do go.

Recently I had a patient return to treatment after about five years. I had seen her and her husband for both couples' marriage therapy and management of his severe, chronic back pain. I had seen them for about a year and he was so doped up on pain killers that he could barely function at all to even participate in the therapy sessions or do any of the homework assignments to help them communicate better. She finally had it and filed for divorce. I hadn't helped them, and his chronic pain, if anything, was worse, and they had dropped out of therapy. They had a child—who was the most important thing in his life—and there was some bitterness over custody, which he lost. I was surprised to learn, from this lady when she returned for treatment, that after the divorce it seemed to wake him up and he started living again and even got remarried and now sees his child on a regular basis. His ex-wife was also doing much better and was returning to treatment for different reasons. So why do I mention this patient? He illustrates the need for a purpose in life. The divorce seemed to make him face reality—before he had just given up—and then he started focusing on what he could do to have a life and have his child in it. He is still in chronic, severe pain but he has somehow, and I give him the credit for doing it, found ways of coping without such overdependence on drugs and with some meaningful purpose in his life.

If you have a skill or knowledge you can teach it to others at community centers for free you will get far more than you give.

Religion/Prayer

I'm not a minister or preacher. I was raised as a Methodist but now I'm more of a pantheist. If religion is important to you and helps you, then use it. Go to church, praise the Lord, and make a joyful noise unto the Lord, and enjoy this day that the Lord has given to you. If praying helps, then by all means pray. If reading scripture works, then by all means read scripture.

Have you heard the story about the man who asks the priest, "Father is it okay to smoke while I pray?"

The priest replies, "Of course not, my son, prayer is a sacrament and should be done in a serious manner."

"Well, father, is it okay to pray while I smoke?"

"Of course my son," says the priest, "prayer is appropriate at any time."

Or, did you hear about the man in Nevada who bought 10 acres of a junkyard? It was a parcel of land no one wanted due to all the junk and was generally considered a very poor piece of property. He worked for several years cleaning it up, planting various desert flowers and cacti, putting in big boulders, and making walking trails with seats under the shade trees. He did such a good job that the place became famous and people would come from hundreds of miles just to see his desert garden.

The man was proud of his work and would greet each visitor after they had toured his garden. One woman, after touring the garden said to him, "You know mister, you have a really beautiful garden, but I think you left something out. You haven't thanked the Lord enough." The man nodded his head and replied, "You know you're right. Without the miracle of life, the soil, the air, sunshine, and rain and all of God's gifts, there wouldn't be much of a garden here. But you should have seen it when He had it all by himself."

One prayer that I recommend to everyone of any or no faith is the Serenity Prayer: "**God grant me the serenity to accept the things that I cannot change, the courage to change the things I can, and the wisdom to know the difference**." If you can change something in your life, do so; if not, let it go. Repeat this prayer daily and live that way and you'll feel better.

What you don't want is coming away from a church service feeling worse, or a preacher who won't listen to you, and/or who tells you to quit doing anything else for your pain and just to pray and read scriptures. It's like the man in the Midwest who was caught in a flood. The water had risen to his front door and a rowboat came by and the rescuers said, "Get in the boat man. The river's going to rise another five to ten feet. You've got to get out of here."

The man replied, "No, I'm staying. I trust in the Lord. He will save me."

Two hours later another rowboat came by and now the waters were up to the second floor and almost to the roof. The man in the boat called to the man leaning out of the second-floor window, "Mister, get in the boat. The water's gonna rise another 6 to 8 feet. You've got to get out of there."

The man replied adamantly, "No. I trust in the Lord. He will save me."

Two hours later the waters had risen so high that the man was seated on the top of his roof. Soon a helicopter hovered overhead and lowered a basket and shouted down through a bull horn, "Hey, mister get in the basket. You've got to evacuate. The river is going to crest in two hours and it will be over you house."

The man continued to adamantly refuse to leave, saying, "I trust in the Lord, He will save me."

The next morning the man is at the Pearly Gates shouting at St. Peter about how angry he was that despite his belief and faith the Lord hadn't saved him. St. Peter said, "Hold on mister. You've got no call to be mad at the Lord. He sent you two rowboats and a helicopter."

The moral of the tale: use what help you can find, religious or otherwise.

Dressing Up

Do you remember playing dress up as a kid and how much fun it was? If not, you missed something fun. When you're depressed and in pain you don't want to do much of anything, let alone dressing up. You tend to hang around in sloppy old house clothes and/or an old bathrobe. If you're a woman you don't bother with makeup and if you're a man you don't shave; it's just too much trouble.

Do it anyway. Take a shower or bath and really enjoy the hot water as you wash your body. Concentrate on enjoying that moment. Wash your hair, dry off with a big clean bath towel, shave and/or put on makeup, and then dress in some nice clothes. Look in the mirror and smile. You'll be amazed at how much better you feel. Then go out, if only for a short walk, or to the mall to walk around. Enjoy.

"I don't want to. It hurts too much and besides it takes me an hour or two just to get it all together. It's just too much." Okay, use one of your guilt-free depression days but then dress up tomorrow. Try it, or not, your choice.

The clothes don't make the man or woman, but they sure do help. If you dress like a bum you'll likely feel like a bum.

Chapter 19:
Constipation

The ugly little secret that they don't really tell you about, constipation—stopped up, can't go. Some people don't have a problem with this, but most people on strong pain medication do. I didn't think that this deserved a whole section by itself, but then, as I thought of it, I decided it did, as no one ever really talks much about it and there is a lot they don't tell you. Again as with all of this, what works for you will have to be a trial and error process.

Did you hear the one about the body parts arguing about who was the most important? The heart says, "I'm most important as, if I don't beat blood doesn't get pumped to all of you and you can't live." The lungs say, "I'm the most important as, if I don't breathe you won't get oxygen and will die." Several other parts make their case and then the brain says, "I'm the most important as I tell all of you what to do." "Oh, shut up," says the anus, "I'm the most important and I can prove it. When I quit working everybody hurts." The anus demonstrated by stopping up and they all quickly agreed he was the most important. Notice I didn't use he/she as everyone knows men are all assholes, so no need to be gender neutral. Supposed to be a little humor there. Laugh. It will make you feel better.

You need to know what your normal cycle of bowel movement is. Are you used to going daily or twice a day or only every other or every third day. Whatever is normal for you, if you go longer than that without a movement, it's time to take a laxative. Don't wait till it gets really bad. You can actually die of an obstructed bowel. Talk to your pharmacist and/or physician about what might be right for you to use.

Read the packaging instructions. You may need to take most laxatives about 24 hours before you get any results from them. If you wait until you're really constipated, it's likely that you're in for a bad 24 hours. I had that happen once and that pain was worse than my back pain. It was like having a broom stick stuck up my ass and I couldn't get it out. I tried

Fleet enemas—where you squirt some liquid up your anus—but couldn't keep the liquid in long enough to do any good. So I suffered, I mean really suffered, for a day until the *Ex-lax* took effect.

There are prescription drugs you can take, but if it is on a weekend or holiday you're out of luck. Since then I have found an over-the-counter product, recommended to me by my MD, that works well, and within several hours rather than 24. It's called *Miralax*. You can also take a daily fiber supplement like *Metamusil*. This has the advantage of adding fiber to your diet, which is supposed to be healthy. But even with this I was still having problems. I never had to worry about this stuff until I started taking all the pain medications. This is one of the reasons why I want to get off of the strong pain medications. Suppositories are good but you can't get them past the anal sphincter with just your finger. You'll need some small blunt object to push it all the way past the sphincter or it won't do any good.

It is one of the few times that you can say, "Shit happens," and be happy about it.

Chapter 20:
Perspective

Keeping it in perspective is another coping strategy that is easy to say but harder to do. The old saying, "I felt sorry for myself because I had no shoes, until I met a man with no feet," illustrates perspective.

Watching all the starving, destitute people all over the world on CNN and the other news programs shows me how fortunate I really am. Even in my own city of Hilo, I can compare myself to many others who don't have electricity or running water and feel how fortunate I am. Perspective is relative, however. A person who doesn't have a high-speed connection to the Internet may be very envious of the person who does and not appreciate that many people don't have any access. A person in severe pain who can walk and talk may not appreciate that he/she is much better off than the person who has severe pain and is confined to a wheelchair. Everything that is, is by comparison.

When you're in severe pain, it doesn't matter that another person is much worse off or that you could be, too. Like the person says, "Don't tell me worrying doesn't do any good. All the things I worry about never happen." Just because I'm better off than many others doesn't mean I'm not in severe pain.

Trying to keep one's pain in perspective is a difficult task. Most of us wouldn't change our problems for someone else's if we knew the depth of their problems. It is hard to walk a mile in someone else's shoes; they just don't fit. I have walked several miles in my own severe pain yet I can't know your pain.

Chapter 21:
More Tools

Massage/Hugs/Creams

A good massage is often a great way to relieve pain at least temporarily. Sometimes it hurts too much to even be touched. Some health insurance will even pay for a therapeutic massage if it is referred by your primary care physician. There are at least a half dozen or more different types of massage and you'll have to try to find which type works for you. If you're fortunate enough to have a spouse or significant other, whether living with you or not, you can get them to give you a massage. There is a whole area of the healing arts just devoted to the healing powers of touch. Google "healing power of touch" and you'll get over 600,000 hits. There is something about being touched in a caring way by another person that is very restful and pleasing. It's best done in a quiet space with soothing music on in the background. Most malls these days have walk-in massages to help relieve the tension of our hectic lives. You might not have the time to schedule a massage for next Tuesday, but you're right there walking by and you can take 10 to 15 minutes for yourself to relax.

It is strange how couples get out of the habit of touching. I routinely recommend that they lovingly give each other a two-to-three-minute foot massage with some hand cream. The couples that actually do it report how wonderful it is both to receive the massage and to give it.

There are also many different types of "healing" creams and lotions. I am skeptical of their claims of miraculous cures for almost anything that ails you. Reminds me of the traveling circus "snake oil" salesman, "Step right up ladies and gentlemen. This product is absolutely, money back, guaranteed to cure backache, headache, upset stomach, ..." If they do work it may be due to the "placebo affect" and that simply put, means that if a person strongly believes that a product will help them, then it probably will, at least to some degree.

Placebo pain pills are just as effective in relieving pain as "real" pain pills—for about 80% of the population—but both the patient and the doctor have to believe that it is a real pain pill or it won't work. Don't you feel better as soon as you walk into your doctor's office? I know I do. It's like we've been conditioned from childhood that doctors make us better, and then the simple act of walking in the doctor's door triggers the mind's expectations that things are going to be better.

Hugs are another great coping strategy. I hug my son and daughter and even my former wife almost every time that I see them and when we part. Hugs are free and they feel good. Ask for them and give them. Google "hug therapy" and you'll get 570,000 plus hits.

Groups

Group therapy is an old and well-used therapeutic approach. The American Chronic-pain Association has a very good and well thought out guide to start your own chronic-pain support/education group. Only people who actually have their own chronic pain are allowed—except for invited speakers—to participate and to lead the groups. Their guidelines are modeled along the lines of Alcoholics Anonymous groups including such things as confidentiality, sponsors, and 10 steps. There are no fees or records involved. They stress that members should focus on what they have found that works for them as coping skills and only minimally talk about their pain per se. In other words, it's not just a bitch and complaint session.

When my own situation improves enough I'll probably try to start such a group in Hilo. In the past when I've tried, there hasn't been enough interest to get even one or two people to come to a meeting. There are plenty of people in my area who have severe pain, but for one reason or another they don't come to a group. Hilo and the surrounding area are very rural and a lot of people can't afford the gas money to come into town for a group meeting. Some say they would come, but don't, and some say they don't want to be around any group whether with others in pain or a group of so-called normal people. I think I'm like that when my pain is bad; I don't want to be around anybody.

Unfortunately, some, most, people don't like groups and would rather have their own individual therapist. Each to his own tastes. For some, groups work great. In a group you don't have to worry about explaining your pain and pacing behavior to the other members, they understand.

Insurance

Hawaii residents are fortunate because the state provides health insurance for almost everyone. But finding a doctor who will take the state-welfare type of insurance is another matter. Even if you're lucky enough to have very good health insurance, on the Big Island it is very hard to find a doctor who is willing to take on new patients. It is to some degree like we are in a third-world country and if you need a specialist, in most cases, you have to go to the main Island Oahu, which means you need to fly, because there are no ferries. We, in Hilo, have one really good pain-management doctor. The experts I saw on Oahu didn't have anything to offer me that my Hilo pain doctor hadn't already done.

I've talked about the mess of the Workman's Compensation insurance elsewhere in this book. But all that said, it's better to have health insurance than not. The drugs alone are so expensive as to be prohibitive without insurance. Most of the insurance companies are not as bad as Workman's Compensation but to get authorization for something like aquatherapy, acupuncture, physical therapy, or a TENS unit, you have to have a doctor whose staff are savvy in the ways of insurance companies and able to follow up on a request or it will take months to get approval.

Insurance companies, like all companies, are in business to make money. That is their primary purpose and they make more by denying coverage of anything they can. They are not in business to help you. They try to sell you their plan by telling you how much they want to help you but make no mistake about it, their primary mission is to make money. And that is not bad. That is the American system. They will gladly take your monthly premium payment but they are not so glad or quick to pay out for expensive treatment if they can find a legitimate way of denying it.

I know some doctors who now work on a cash or check basis only and won't take any insurance. They will send a bill into the insurance company so that you can get reimbursed whatever the insurance company is willing to pay. The insurance companies are making millions of dollars but they often don't pay enough for the doctor to stay in business. In the same vein, there are some people who are choosing to go without insurance at all.

Enough. I can feel myself getting tense and I don't want to go there.

Heat/Ice

Heat and cold are some of the oldest forms of treatment for pain and are still very effective. When I first tried a heating pad on my back I didn't think it did any good. Now I love putting a rolled-up towel under my heating pad—placed so that it will be in the lower lumbar area—and a towel on top of the heating pad and then lie on my back and enjoy the heat.

I've tried the frozen ice packs but they don't seem to work for me. You need to try both and decide what works best for you.

TENS

TENS stands for "transcutaneous electrical neural stimulation." There are many different types of TENS devices. The most common ones that are portable are about the size of a pack of cigarettes and the unit is clipped onto your belt or shirt or blouse. The nurse at you doctor's office will show you how to use them. I was happy to have the unit. I put the patches on my lower back, Heaven. What it feels like is not a shock but like thousands of fingernails scratching lightly but very rapidly in the pain area.

TrueBack

I've already described this in my "On-Going Journey" part of this book. I just wanted to mention it again as one of the best coping tools I have found. You can check it out on the web by googling *Trueback*, and you'll see a picture and description as well as sources for purchase.

Homeopathy

I don't know much about this one but I'm trying to cover most all the bases here and I know some people take this approach and find it useful. It is defined in *The American Heritage Dictionary* as: "A system for treating disease based on the administration of minute doses of a drug that in massive amounts produces symptoms in healthy individuals similar to those of the disease itself." I have heard that there are some good homeopathic doctors who really help people who haven't been helped by more traditional medical practices. Ask questions and check out the credentials of the person you're seeing. Don't just blindly trust someone, whether it's a homeopathic doctor or a traditional medical doctor.

Acupuncture

Acupuncture has been used for thousands of years in Chinese and Asian countries. It is now coming into the mainstream of medicine in America. It is covered by some health insurance companies and Workman's Compensation. I've described my encounter with it in my "On-Going Journey" earlier in this book. Even though I'm not currently doing it, I would recommend you give it a try, but first discuss it with your medical doctor and check out the credentials of whomever you go to see. If I don't continue to get better on my own current treatment program, I will return to this option. Many of my patients have told me of very beneficial results they have obtained from it. I did return and saw another acupuncturist for five sessions but I wasn't getting any better so I quit.

Screaming/Crying/Moaning

When the anger and frustrations build up, sometimes breathing and changing your self-talk just isn't enough. It's okay to scream and holler and curse. Curse God and everything. Shout it as loud as you can. But, choose a private place to do this kind of venting. Don't do it in front of children, or friends, or family, or anyone. It's very unpleasant for someone else to listen to. So go out to the seaside, or in the woods, or somewhere where no one can hear you and let it all out for about 10 to 15 minutes. It works. I have one lady who gets in her car—about once every few months—and closes all the windows and just screams and shouts and pounds on the steering wheel. I've suggested she do this when she is parked someplace away from people and not while driving.

Once you've let out the steam of anger, you may be okay for several days or weeks. This is not for everyone, but it does seem to help some people, and since they are going to end up doing it anyway, I think it's better to plan it so you do it away from other people.

Crying is another good release and again is best done in private so as to not distress others. You feel better after a good cry. If you find yourself doing it often in front of others, you might want to consider: (1) trying some antidepressant medication, and/or (2) asking yourself if you're doing it to get attention and sympathy, and/or (3) addressing it in psychotherapy.

Moaning is another way of expressing your hurt. I use this one, often saying—when I get up from sitting especially—"Uh, oh, ah, uuuhh, oah, oooh." I call it my "oh, ah meter" going off. Some people are moaners and some aren't. For those of us who are it seems to help relieve the pain just to be able to let it out vocally. Again however, it's not so pleasant for others to hear. I also make noises at pleasurable times, like during sex, or eating something that tastes good, I do lots of uhm, mum good; these are pleasure moans.

Some people find that beating a pillow, physical exercise to the extent they can, cleaning the refrigerator, throwing rocks out to sea, or chopping wood also helps relieve the tension. Of course you pay the price if you do physical things that you know will later cause you pain.

Writing

You can keep a journal in the manner I explained under the "Anger/Emotional Management" section of this book. Or you can just write in a paper journal or on your computer. By writing it down it seems to be a way of getting the thoughts and feelings that are bothering you out of your brain so that you don't have to be bothered with them.

The writing doesn't have to be in any particular format and you don't have to worry about spelling or grammar. You can free associate and write anything that comes to your mind. It doesn't have to make sense. You can write swear words over and over, filling page after page until you're tired of it. It's for you and no one else has to see it. There are even books on writing therapy.

Several of my patients find it a useful way to deal with bad dreams and/or conscious thoughts. Write them down and then burn the paper up, symbolically getting rid of them. They may come back but you can always get rid of them again.

What does this have to do with pain? It's another way of relieving stress, which causes tension, which makes your pain worse. Are you getting the message yet?

Try it. See if it works for you.

Helping Others/Volunteering

Helping others is a great way to deal with your own pain. I do this when I do psychotherapy with my patients: helping them helps me. During the time that you are helping others—visiting patients in the hospital or nursing homes, taking someone for a ride, whatever—you're not thinking about your own pain and problems and there is the feeling of accomplishment in helping someone else, even if it is in some minor way.

There are all kinds of ways to volunteer to help others. You can read to others in the library or help others learn English as a second language, help out at your local church, learn to be a docent at a local museum or cultural center, or see what you might be able to do at a seniors' center. The nice thing about volunteering is that you can set the amount of time, one or two hours, and days, once a week, when you will be able to volunteer. You don't get paid in money but you get rewarded well with the satisfaction of good human interaction.

Volunteering can also be a step towards getting back to work, just getting very gradually used to being somewhere else for a few hours a day, a few days a week. If you have been out of work from a traditional 9 to 5 type of job for two or more years, you have to give your body and mind time to gradually get back into the daily routine of work.

Steven W. Pollard, PhD

Family/Friends

It almost goes without saying that family and friends are very important, but we often only pay lip service to them. You need to put your money where your mouth is. Actually spend time with them on a regular basis, but don't be afraid to set boundaries about what you can and can't do. Just because you're not working—a paying job—due to your injury and pain, doesn't mean they can dump the kids on you every day or expect you to do the things for them that you can't even do for yourself, like shopping and/or cooking. Just taking care of yourself and all of your own appointments and paperwork pertaining to your injury is a full-time job—you just don't get paid much to do it.

It is hard to do but you need to learn how to ask family and friends for help. You don't want to impose on them, so you ask them in a way that lets them know that it is okay if they say, "No, I can't do that at this time." That's okay, you've respected them by saying in advance that it would be okay if they say no. Most of the time they will say yes if they can, as you would say yes to them if the situation were reversed and they were the one in severe pain asking for help.

"Yes but I don't want to bother them, they have their own lives and . . ." Okay go ahead and suffer, you're allowed. It is a difficult balancing act to not ask too often for help. If you ask too much they may build up resentment and start avoiding you. On the other hand, if you don't ask for help when you really need it, you not only further isolate yourself, but you deny others the pleasure of letting them help you.

Family Meetings

Whether or not you are in severe pain, having regular family meetings—at least once a week or once a month—is a good idea. It can be done at supper time, or breakfast, or whenever the family members agree. That is a time for each person to say what their thoughts or feelings are about a particular problem or situation, without blaming, but rather looking for solutions that are practical and agreeable with everyone.

Family calendars are also a good idea for keeping track of who is doing what, when, and where. My extended family does this on computers on the Internet, so that even though we don't all live together we can post things to the family calendar to let others know what we're doing.

These meetings are a way of communication that helps to avoid unnecessary hurt feelings. And by keeping the stress down in the family it does what? Say it with me, "Keeps my stress down which helps lessen my pain."

Communication/Relationships

Scientists who study communication say that only something like 15% of communication is based on actual content of the spoken words. Most communication is from body movement, facial expression, eye movements, tone, and pacing of voice. You can say the same thing and mean the opposite depending on inflection and emphasis. Try saying "I love you," and meaning it and then "I love you," and meaning the opposite. Do it in front of a mirror.

Good communication is critical for good relationships. **Good relationships reduce stress and help keep your pain lower.** I give the following information to almost all my patients whether they are in severe physical pain or not.

Relationship Building and Maintenance

Having a good relationship with a significant other or even friends requires desire, work, and commitment. There are no guarantees and it does take two to want to build and maintain the relationship whether it is a love relationship or a friendship. People and relationships change over time. Some of the items below apply to just a love relationship and some apply equally to both a love-type relationship as well as to a friend relationship.

Wanting a good love relationship: **critical requirement**. Some people don't really want a relationship, but rather just someone to have sex with or someone to do things for them (cook and clean, fix the car, etc.). This is okay if you both agree to this type of relationship, but it is very rare that this type of relationship lasts; one or the other person begins to feel used and ends the relationship.

Shared values, interests, and goals: **critical requirement**. Over time, if you have very different values, interests, and goals you may grow apart and not have enough basis for a relationship. Do you both want an equal relationship? You need to discuss these areas with your partner.

Commitment: critical requirement. Wanting to have a good relationship is not going to make it happen by itself, any more than wanting to have a million dollars will make you a millionaire. Both of you have to commit to doing the work, **on a regular basis**, that is required to have a good relationship.

Conflict resolution: critical requirement. Common areas of conflict: communication style, money management, chores, parenting, relatives, time management, and sex. If you cannot or are not able (for whatever reason—no blame) to resolve the significant conflicts in your relationship, you can still use these tools to have an ending of the relationship in as friendly a manner as possible.

Love and liking: these issues are often **critically important**. The definition of love varies greatly for each individual. The definition and meaning of love needs to be discussed and agreed upon. You may love someone but can't live with them, or you may like them but not love them. Liking the other person is a major part of the glue that holds a relationship together. You may love someone but if you don't like them, it may be very difficult to be in a relationship with the person.

Trust and honesty: critical elements in a relationship. Trust is given by trusting the other person, and earned by doing what you say you are going to do. Most people place great value on honesty, and it is required to have a truly meaningful relationship. Honesty, like trust, is given and earned by being truthful and not deceiving or lying directly or by omission.

Dignity and respect: critical requirement. Both parties in the relationship need to feel that they are being treated with dignity and respect.

Bottom line: decide what is the **absolute minimum you absolutely must have** from your partner to stay in the relationship. If you're getting that, consider letting the rest of the stuff you don't like (your complaints) go. They're not big enough to end the relationship, so let them go. Accept and enjoy what you have and/ or negotiate for changes in the smaller things to meet each other's needs.

Tools: to use to build and maintain a good relationship.

Rules of Engagement: for intimate relationships to discuss problems or disagreements.

1. Remember that the purpose is to build the relationship, not to prove who is right; keep reminding yourself of this.
2. Don't try to engage in discussion when drunk or high (can be drunk on anger or hurt—see below).
3. Set a time, place, and agenda that is mutually agreeable.
4. No violence or threats of violence allowed, no cursing, and no yelling. If any of this occurs stop the meeting for that session. You may want to use a tape recorder to make both of you aware that what you are saying is being recorded and monitored. The purpose of the recorder is not to prove who said what, but to make both parties be more polite, since they know it is being recorded.
5. Take a deep breath to relax, time out, or cool down if either party gets too emotionally upset.
6. Use "I" messages and "active listening"; see below.
7. Weekly management meeting required.

8. Agree to disagree about perceptions of the past, to avoid the never-ending cycle of arguing about who said and/or did what. "You said/did . . ." "Did not." "Did too." "Did not." No negative comments or put downs about the other person in any way, including teasing, which can too easily be used to justify a hurtful comment, "I was just teasing." Stop it. It doesn't help and makes communication harder.

9. Use a problem-solving process to reach solutions to problems, not to place blame or prove who's right.

Active listening: the goal is for you and your partner to both feel that the other person understands you. As with a relationship in general, you have to **really want to listen** to understand the other person's point of view. If either of you feel misunderstood, you aren't doing this part correctly. Biggest blocks to listening: arguing, trying to win, or prove the other person wrong, or prove yourself right. Being angry. You might try using the format that follows to develop your active listening skills.

1. Paraphrase what you heard the other person say. Include the feelings behind the message, not just the words. Include your

interpretation of the words, e.g. "Let me see if I got what you're saying . . ." It is not sufficient to say, "I understand what you're saying." You may think you do and you may be right, but unless you openly express your understanding of what you think the other person said, you wouldn't know if you got it right or wrong.

2. Ask, "Is that right?" If the person says "No," don't say "Yes it is, that's what you said." Say, "I must have misunderstood. Please tell me again." If the person says "Yes," you can go to number 3, if they say "No," then you have to go back to number 1.

3. Ask, "May I reply?" If the other person says, "No," let the other person go on. If the other person says, "Yes," the other person is agreeing to now be quiet, and listen to you using the same format.

"I" messages: the purpose of "I" messages is to communicate an area of concern or problem to a significant other in a way that is less likely to be perceived as an attack (not blaming the other person) and to take responsibility for your thoughts, feelings, actions, and needs.

Format: is something like this: "Honey, I have a problem. I care about our relationship and I would like to speak with you about my problem with (fill in the blank e.g. anger, chores around the house, money management, intimacy, handling the kids, etc.). I want my needs to be met in this area and I want to meet your needs. Can we set a time to talk about this?"

Example:

"You" message: most people use "you" messages, which tend to be perceived as an attack or blame. "You always leave a mess around the house. Why can't you ever clean up after yourself? You never listen to me. You treat me like dirt."

Subtle "you" message (still blaming while pretending not to): "I have a problem when you leave a mess around the house; when you don't listen to me, etc."

"I" message: "I have a problem. I would like speak with you. I care about our relationship and I don't want to cause any hard feelings. Can we set a time when we can talk about chores around the house? My problem is that I want a neat house and I want to meet your needs in this area so that both you and I feel comfortable with the neatness level of our home."

"I" messages are generally longer than "you" messages in order to fully express your feelings and concerns about a problem area. At the same time you are trying not to blame the other person for your problem. You are letting the other person know that you care about their opinion on the subject and that you are not saying it has to be "my way or the highway."

Anger card: quick reference to help you manage your anger. You can't communicate if you're drunk on anger or hurt.

1. Take a few really deep breaths, exhaling slowly, and tell yourself to relax. It is much more difficult to be angry/hurt if you are relaxed and a slow deep breath is a very good, quick way to relax.

2. Time out/cool downs—think down: who is making you angry/hurt? You. How do you do that? By telling yourself negative things about the situation or person, e.g. "It's not fair. He/she doesn't care about me. She/he is putting me down." Who can make you calm? You. How do you do that? By countering all of the negative self-talk, e.g. "Fair or not, I'm not going to continue to make myself angry or be hurt over this because then I won't be able to listen or communicate. She/he does care about me. And saying he/she doesn't, only helps me justify my anger/hurt. Even if he/she is putting me down, I'm going to take a deep

breath and calm down and not continue to make myself angry about any put downs, intended or not." Cool downs need to last as long as it takes to think down to a calm level. To help in understanding the thinking that continues your anger, finish this sentence, "I'm angry because . . ." Anything you say after "because" is self-talk and that self-talk is what you need to change if you are going to change your feelings about any given situation.

3. Wear a rubber band around your wrist and pull it back and snap the inside of your wrist to remind you that your anger is hurting you—and your partner—and it is up to you to stop it.

Problem solving: critical tool, but it can only be used **after** you have used "I" messages and active listening long enough so that you both feel your point of view is understood by the other. The only way to achieve this level of communication is for each person to ask the other person, "Do you feel that I understand what you're saying?" If the answer from both is "Yes", then, and only then may you constructively go on to the next step of problem solving. If the answer to the question was "No" by either party, then you need to start over. During the problem-solving steps you need to continue to use active listening and I messages.

Steps in the problem-solving process, while using "I" messages and active listening are:

1. Identify the problem. Define its parameters and whose problem it is. Not whose fault it is.
2. Brainstorm as many solutions/coping strategies as possible. Brainstorming means coming up with any ideas you can think of no matter how silly or unworkable they seem. These silly ideas may trigger workable solutions. Put downs and/or sarcasm gets you off track and back to fighting.
3. Evaluate each possible solution. What would be the outcome of each one? Again, no judgments or put-downs. You're not in a court of law trying to prove who's right. If that's what you want, go see an attorney.
4. Based on your evaluation, choose what seems to be the best solution/coping strategy.
5. Agree to try and use and practice the solution during the next week or until your next meeting.
6. If during the practice week you find that the solution you chose is not working for one

or both of you, you need to go back to your list of possible solutions/coping strategies and choose the next best one.

Courting/positive interactions: critical requirement. Both partners need to say and/or do 5 to 10 positive things (saying what you like about the other person or thanking them or complimenting them) a day. You need to return to the positive behaviors of courting, calling each other, doing small things to let the other know you are thinking of them, plan, and go on dates.

Bottom line: both partners need to set specific boundaries that if crossed, will signal the termination of the relationship. These boundaries need to be specific and from your point of view, final. If the other person crosses this boundary, then you may want to do counseling to end the relationship in as amicable a way as possible.

This process of relationship building and maintenance is very difficult and is like learning a new language or building a beautiful garden. The more you work at it and practice it, the easier it gets and the better you get at maintaining your relationship.

Parenting

I'm not going to say a lot about this because there are a lot of good books about parenting. Get them. Read them. Do as instructed. Many families have the same fights every morning getting ready for school, and/or at night getting ready for bed, and/or about doing homework and chores, about getting along with siblings. It's crazy. In fact one definition of insanity is doing the same thing over and over and expecting different results.

If there is excessive stress in the family, it makes you tense, and the more tense you are, the worse your pain is. There will always be some stresses in parenting—or living for that matter—but you can drastically reduce the amount of stress if you know how to communicate and parent effectively and you are thereby reducing or helping to keep your pain at lower levels.

Chapter 22:
Returning to Work

If you are fortunate enough to be able to return to work, please do so very slowly, especially if you've been out of work for an extended period of time. Going back to work is hard. The longer you're out of work, the less likely it is that you will be able to go back. That doesn't mean it's impossible, just less likely.

Your primary care physician is the gatekeeper and the person who can set the standards under which you can go back to work. So you need to present your case to your primary care physician to have your return to work not only for light duty, but to phase yourself back into the routine of getting up and going back to work on a gradually increasing basis. I'd suggest starting with one to two hours a day, two to three days a week, and if you tolerate that okay, then after about a month go to three to four hours a day, three to four days a week, and then in a month if you tolerate that okay go to four to six hours a day, four to five days a week for a month, and so on, until you get back to 8 hours a day. If during any of this process you're in moderate to severe pain, do not hesitate to call your MD and say you can't handle it. The "no pain, no gain" adage doesn't apply here. Pay attention to your pain. If I had I wouldn't be in as much pain as I was. I kept re-injuring myself in small doses. So, don't do as I do, do as I say.

This process of going back to work very slowly may seem very tedious, but it is a lot easier to speed things up once you start back to work than it is to slow it down.

You may think this is too slow and many doctors routinely—it seems without really thinking about it—start a worker off at four hours a day five days a week, and in a month, back to full time. It takes a lot of time to recondition your mind and body to all the rigors of getting back into the "work" routine. Well, for what it's worth, that's my opinion of how best to make a successful transition back to work. Both the employer and worker are often too eager to get back to full time and the worker ends up getting re-injured—not on purpose—but because they push themselves too hard.

Acceptance

What happens if you can't go back to work? That is the BIG question. Helping you get to the stage of acceptance with your pain and altered life is where the rubber hits the road. You may never be able to do all, or even some of the things you could before the injury or illness. In many ways, your life may be very much worse, but if you're willing to work at changing yourself and your attitudes then, in many ways, your life can be better and more meaningful and fulfilling than before the injury. I'm not saying this is easy; it's the hardest thing you'll ever have to do because it requires relentless work and vigilance to avoid old patterns of thinking and behaving.

You may never be able to go back to your old job, but you may be able to learn new skills and find a new job, though it will probably not pay as much. That is another one of those things you need to accept. Getting mad isn't going to change it. That just makes your life worse.

You may be able to go back to school. Vocational Rehabilitation Services (VRS) should be available to you. VRS may be very beneficial in this process of trying to find something you might like and then providing the training needed for you to get into another profession. Unfortunately—there seems to be a lot of use of the word unfortunately in my presentation in this book—there are many VRS workers who just want you to go out and apply for a certain number of jobs each week, regardless of whether or not your doctor is even willing to release you to return to work. The VRS people are only going to get paid if they have you doing something that looks like it will be able to get you back to work.

Chapter 23:
Heroes

So who are the heroes? The doctors who strive to help you? The few who recover and go back to their normal lives? Me? No not me.

To me the real "heroes" are the millions of people who continue to struggle with severe, chronic pain on a daily basis. Yet they keep on going with their lives, helping themselves and others as best they can. They get up every day and do one more day at a time, despite the pain. The heroes are also the families and friends who stand by and support their loved one who is in so much pain, knowing that there is not much that they can do to help them. The heroes are the ones who keep hope and keep on trying.

Feel free to contact me with questions and/or comments at: ChronicPain123@gmail.

com. I will not answer hate mail. I welcome constructive criticism. I'm sure I've made some mistakes and left some things out and probably offended some. If you don't like what I've written, I'm sorry for your loss.

If you did get something useful for yourself out of this book, pass it on to someone else.

To all I say, "Good night and good luck."

Steve

Resources

1. Yourself
2. Your family and friends
3. Doctors and other professionals
4. The American Pain Association
5. The Internet

Things I've learned in no particular order paraphrased and/or quoted from Latitudes & Attitudes.

1. Don't put off what you can do now; waiting is just an illusion.
2. If you ask for things nicely you may get more that wasn't even offered.
3. Even the best of days may have their dark side so be aware.

4. Though your course may appear erratic you are making progress. Daily positive affirmation does help.

5. Don't envy others who seem better off as they have their own problems and you have all you can handle now.

6. Doing the thing you sometimes don't want to is necessary to reach your goals.

7. External things may appear to have changed but they are the same; it is you who has changed.

8. Techknowledge is great but you still have to do the work.

9. The good things are up hill; giving up is ever present but giving up slows your progress.

10. Bliss often comes after disappointment; look for it.

11. Changing directions repeatedly may be necessary to make progress.

12. Though the pain may be chaotic you may find a pattern you can use.

13. Despite the intensity of the pain you may be able to find a safe haven to suffer less.

14. Conserving your energy and staying hydrated is always good.

15. There is no benefit in getting angry or mad at your perceived lack of progress especially when the pain is severe.

16. The scariest journeys may take you to the most beautiful places.
17. Never trust the medical tests and reports, find out for yourself.
18. Stay as alert as you can; there are always hidden dangers you may fall into.
19. Pain sometimes comes in waves, to guess their next occurrence. We may not be able to resist trying to change their course but we can learn to ride with them.

If you're interested in abstract art check out my web site www.abstract-art-wow.com.

I've also written my first novel—the one that got all of my severe back problems started—a Psychosexual Thriller, Erotic, Romance; "Dangerous Deceptive Webs." It should be available at Amazon.com.